Atlas of Vaginal Surgery
Volume 1

Volume 1

Atlas of Vaginal Surgery

Surgical Anatomy and Technique

by

PROF. DR. GÜNTHER REIFFENSTUHL

Director, Frauenklinik, Salzburg, Austria

and

PROF. DR. WERNER PLATZER

Director, Anatomischen Institutes der Universität, Innsbruck, Austria

ILLUSTRATED BY FRANZ BATKE, VIENNA, AUSTRIA

TRANSLATED BY E. JUDITH FRIEDMAN AND EMANUEL A. FRIEDMAN

edited by

EMANUEL A. FRIEDMAN, M.D., Med. Sc.D.

Professor of Obstetrics and Gynecology, Harvard Medical School;
Obstetrician-Gynecologist-in-Chief, Beth Israel Hospital, Boston

1975   W. B. SAUNDERS COMPANY • Philadelphia • London • Toronto

W. B. Saunders Company: West Washington Square
Philadelphia, PA 19105

12 Dyott Street
London, WC1A 1DB

833 Oxford Street
Toronto, Ontario M8Z 5T9, Canada

Title of the original German language edition:
Die vaginalen Operationen
© 1974 Urban and Schwarzenberg, Munich, Germany.
Illustration rights held by Urban and Schwarzenberg.

Atlas of Vaginal Surgery

Vol. I: ISBN 0-7216-7543-3
Vol. II: ISBN 0-7216-7544-1

Last digit is the print number: 9   8   7   6   5   4   3   2

FOREWORD

This splendid atlas of gynecologic surgery encompasses the spectrum of vaginal procedures as practiced and taught in the Austrian school. Not since the highly prized Ferguson translation of the masterful Peham and Amreich classic, long out of print, has there been a book of such stature available on this subject in English.

Those among us who were raised, professionally speaking, in the shadow of the descendants of the great Austrian gynecologic surgeons have had the vicarious reward of that association by exposure to and acquisition of some of the technical skills described herein. The refinements relating to delicate tissue handling and anatomical dissection more than adequately compensate for the extra effort needed to learn these methods and to become proficient in them. Too many American gynecologists have been content with a less satisfactory, albeit acceptable, approach, despite the fact that they are clearly capable of better by virtue of their inherent talents. This work should prove especially useful to them and, although it cannot substitute for first-hand exposure by demonstrations of and participation in dissection techniques in the operating theater under the aegis of an excellent teacher, it can offer them new insights and skills that will benefit their patients.

Perusing this work, the reader will immediately recognize the overriding value of its magnificent illustrations. They reflect the exceptional talent, the many years of intensive experience and the comprehensive grasp of the field possessed by the renowned master artist, Franz Batke, to whom they are a tribute. Nowhere in our current gynecological literature are there drawings of equal caliber insofar as their lucidity, power, realism and accuracy are concerned. They ably serve to infuse life into the text by personalizing details of anatomy and of surgical technique, bringing the reader right into the dissection room and the operating theater where he can study and assimilate the lessons they teach.

Of equivalent importance, moreover, is the complementary textual material. The authors have provided keen insights into the philosophy and art that has characterized the Austrian gynecological heritage. The profusion of detail, albeit not meant for cursory or superficial reading, will prove to be of immense value to the serious student, particularly where it deals with the orchestration of the surgical team. This special emphasis is unique among surgical atlases, which, heretofore, have concentrated almost exclusively on the surgeon's activities in performing the sequential steps of the procedures. Experienced gynecologists are well aware that the assistants play a major role in the execution of operative surgery, most especially in those operations done by the vaginal route, where the luxuries of ample exposure and accessibility are often severely constrained.

Additionally, integration has been achieved between anatomical information and surgical principles. The section on pelvic anatomy by Professor Platzer is at once complete and limited, presenting a comprehensive review of surgically relevant and useful material, yet avoiding the temptation to expound in depth on the type of minutiae that concern the anatomist—but are decried by the clinician. Sound anatomical knowledge is, of course, the foundation of good surgical practice; without it, technical skills are valueless. The emphasis given here, therefore, is appropriate, and the gynecologic surgeon, even if of seasoned experience, would be well advised to take full advantage of this exposition to learn or to review pelvic anatomy.

Professor Reiffenstuhl, whose surgical skills and work on the pelvic lymphatics are well known and admired, has built upon the anatomical foundation of the first section to provide a thorough discourse on the operative steps involved in those vaginal procedures that are being done, and, as a consequence, have been tested and perfected in his hands. The accumulated experience and wise surgical judgment that he brings to the task are everywhere apparent, especially in his discussions of the problems the surgeon is likely to encounter if he ignores some seemingly insignificant detail or alters a sequence of steps. There is a refreshing honesty inherent in the recurrent disclosures of errors, through which he has learned (thus alerting us) to avoid similar costly mistakes.

Like its predecessors, this book does not try to present a compendium of all vaginal procedures. The authors have confined themselves only to procedures with which they have had extensive experience. This approach has the advantage of ensuring the reader that each detail has the weight of authority and embodies refinements of technique based on a distillation of that experience. In sum, we can say the book is monumental. It represents the combined expertise and singular talents of an anatomist, a surgeon and an artist—to yield a reference source that will be invaluable to the novice as well as to the experienced gynecologic surgeon.

EMANUEL A. FRIEDMAN, M.D., SC.D.

PREFACE

The prerequisites for a successful surgical practice are talent and education. One is born with the first. Technical details can be learned, but must be developed by conscientious schooling. Indispensable for independent execution of surgical procedures are the intimate knowledge of anatomy and the experience garnered from association with and exposure to a teacher who operates along typical lines.

The German literature contains exemplary instructional material in gynecologic surgery based on the collective wealth of experience of its authors. Such material warrants primacy in the libraries of every practicing gynecologist. This notwithstanding, we undertook to create a new work on this subject in 1965. Our objective was not directed at providing something better than heretofore available, but rather, it originated with our concept and desire to elucidate the anatomic surgical principles that we have developed and tested in the course of evolving our large experience. Our aim was to coordinate this material in a uniform and comprehensively detailed manner.

In scope, this book is meant to serve in providing technical advice for carrying out vaginal surgical procedures. The exclusive preference for the vaginal approach in our discussion here is based on the philosophy that the gynecologist must become proficient in these techniques and that he should practice them extensively.

For each gynecologic disorder, there are a number of available operations. To have concerned ourselves with all of them in the same detail as with those that we prefer would have expanded the scope of this volume excessively. We concur with Frisch, who stated in the preface to his atlas of surgical gynecology, that "it is better to learn one good method than to recapitulate all methods that have been recommended over the course of the decade." For the same reason, we have avoided any critical mention of the relevant literature so as not to disturb the uniformity and flow of the total picture.

Vaginal operations were consciously preselected for presentation on the basis of preferences engendered by their origin in the Austrian school and the fact that they have been retained in our surgical armamentarium to date. If this volume is slanted subjectively by a systematic representation of personally developed operative techniques, then our purpose has been realized in helping to disseminate knowledge concerning those vaginal operative procedures that are practiced extensively at one author's clinic. It should reflect the art of surgery as currently practiced by the Austrian gynecologist, and as it has always been practiced.

Even though we admit that we have not defended the views of our teachers of anatomy and of gynecology in all matters, we do believe it is the duty of the pious scholar toward his forebears to mention them in gratitude: von Hayek, Pernkopf, Antoine and Navratil.

In dividing our material, we portrayed first the anatomic conditions, and then built upon this information to describe the various operative methods.

In our operative descriptions, details were presented that were deemed necessary for purposes of reducing the hazards of each procedure. Additionally, the activities of both assisting physicians were delved into in great detail because experience has taught us that cooperative contributions by assistants is essential for the success of vaginal surgery. The surgeon must not only have full command of the operative details of the procedure itself, but he must be able to instruct his assistants systematically. Only in this way can the interplay of all three operating physicians be achieved and transmit to the observer the feeling of facility and smoothness. If well orchestrated, the procedure can be shortened considerably.

Furthermore, we have set out to show the hazards of the operations, as presented to both beginner and more advanced surgeon, when they falter. Trepidation alone, although yielding much discomfiture, is not a good advisor. It is far better, therefore, for us to explain as frankly as possible what we and others have observed as errors and dangers in performing vaginal surgery. Every surgeon who is dedicated to the operative approach has suffered many technical setbacks, but not everyone is prepared to acknowledge them.

At the beginning, an anatomical introduction is presented. It consists of a summation based on discourses dealing with individual regions as viewed from the surgeon's vantage. We chose this approach, rather than the more orthodox anatomical compartmentalization, which is not applicable to surgical practice, because it seemed to be a requisite for the operative section that follows.

Along similar lines, it appeared to be necessary to present sketches of the different operative steps to point out specific, important anatomical details. Special care has been devoted to these illustrations by virtue of the value we ascribe to them as an integral complement to the text of a surgical atlas. All anatomical illustrations were produced from specimens prepared at the Anatomischen Institut der Universität Innsbruck, through the invaluable aid of

Dr. Maurer and others. We wish to thank them here heartily. In particular, we wish to point out that all semischematic and schematic illustrations were drawn from original specimens. Illustrations of the clinical aspects were all based on observations made in the course of actual procedures done on live patients. In order to achieve the special characteristics of naturalness in these figures, thousands of colored stereoscopic photographs were taken during the operations. These then served as models for the illustrations. Not one was made from memory or reproduced from previously published pictures. The stereophotographic technique has permitted the artist to grasp the correct depth of the particular operative field, and to represent it accurately.

All the drawings were created by the academic artist, Franz Batke, with whom the authors have been associated for purposes of cooperative activities dealing with several books for more than 25 years. Franz Batke is an artist recognized by American medical illustrators as one of the best illustrators of anatomical atlases and surgical textbooks. He has brought to this book not only his decades of experience, but also his personal and amicable relationships with both authors. He has worked on this volume with obvious gratification. For the illustrations contained herein, which represent ten years of carefully detailed work, we owe considerable thanks to Franz Batke.

Aid in providing the stereophotography during surgery was given by surgical nurse, Erasta Jagerhofer, who is very knowledgeable, always friendly and cooperative, and willing to sacrifice much time and effort in our behalf. For all this, we are very appreciative.

For reading and correcting the anatomical section, we thank the assistants, Drs. R. Putz and S. Poisel of the Anatomische Institut Innsbruck. In editorially correcting the clinical part, Dr. Staudach, of the Frauenklinik Salzburg, has provided a great deal of support for which we are particularly grateful.

To our publishers, M. Urban of Munich and his father, Dr. Heinz Urban, who edited and produced the German edition of this book, we offer very special thanks. Dr. Müller, the scientfic coworker of the publisher, who always demonstrated great understanding of this work, and Mr. Gullath, who managed the production, were both instrumental in ensuring that the book would appear in its present form.

G. REIFFENSTUHL AND W. PLATZER

CONTENTS

ANATOMICAL DESCRIPTION

EXTERNAL GENITALIA

The external female genitalia (Fig. 1), more specifically the vulva, consists of the labia majora, the labia minora, the clitoris, the vaginal vestibule and the mons pubis. Lying in close apposition in nulliparas are the labia majora, which border on the pudendal aperture. The vaginal vestibule is exposed only when the labia are parted.

Laterally, the *labia majora* are separated from the genitofemoral sulci by lateral depressions and the interconnecting gluteoperineal tissues. The genitofemoral sulcus borders the vulva, perineum and anus posterolaterally and continues anteriorly into the inguinal sulcus and posteriorly into the gluteal sulcus. Medially to the genitofemoral sulcus, an accessory groove is sometimes found beginning in the urogenital region (laterally to the labia majora) and ending in the gluteal region. The two labia come together in the midline at the anterior labial commissure that borders on the mons pubis inferiorly. Toward the perineum, one finds the posterior labial commissure, which seems to separate the vaginal vestibule from the sharp-edged labial frenulum (frenulum labiorum pudendi). On their outer surface, the labia majora are covered with pigmented skin that contains numerous sebaceous and sweat glands, as well as nerve endings and hair follicles.

Subcutaneously within the labia majora are sheets of connective tissue that collectively form the corpus fibrosum. Adipose tissue may penetrate between these connective tissue layers from the mons pubis as well as from the perineum. Smooth muscle fibers can be found also in variable numbers. The connective tissue layer radiates into the perineal body (see p. 8) at one end and into the abdominal subcutaneous tissue at the other. The deep clitoral ligament (ligamentum fundiforme clitoridis) arises approximately in the middle of the mons pubis. The uterine round ligament (ligamentum teres, ligamentum rotunda uteri) radiates subcutaneously upward bilaterally from each inguinal canal (see p. 67).

Figure 1.

External female genitalia, showing the underlying bony pelvis. *1* Labium majus, *2* genitofemoral sulcus, *3* gluteoperineal area, *4* accessory sulcus, *5* ischial tuberosity (palpable bony prominence), *6* ischial spine, *7* anterior labial commissure, *8* posterior labial commissure, *9* labium minus, *10* frenulum clitoridis, *11* frenulum labiorum pudendi, *12* urethral papilla and ostium of the external urethra, *13* frenulum praeputii, *14* glans clitoridis.

2

See illustration on opposite page.

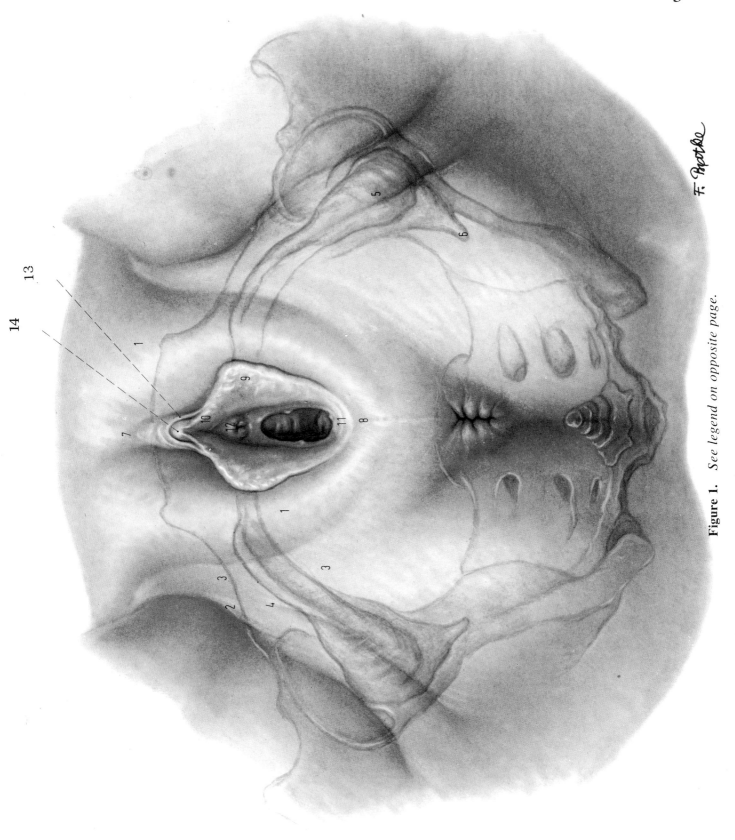

Figure 1. *See legend on opposite page.*

The *labia minora,* also called nymphae, border medially on the vaginal vestibule and are separated laterally from the labia majora by the nympholabial sulci. They separate cranially into medial and lateral components. The medial part is the clitoral frenulum that extends to the underside of the glans clitoridis, while the more laterally-located preputial frenulum forms the clitoral prepuce. The labia minora become smaller in their caudal extension and become apposed to each other immediately in front of the posterior labial commissure above the pudendal frenulum, a diagonal skinfold. This frenulum is sometimes inaccurately attributed to the labia majora.

The labia minora are free of hair and are covered only by a thin layer of cornified squamous epithelium. They contain mostly elastic fibers, blood vessels and nerves as well as coarse connective tissue. In addition, they possess sebaceous glands but no sweat glands. They develop to different sizes, but are usually hidden by the labia majora. They can, however, protrude from between the labia majora, and may actually even extend a considerable distance (as in the so-called Hottentot apron).

The vaginal introitus and the urethral meatus open into the vaginal vestibule between the labia minora. On either side of the introitus are the openings of the ducts of Bartholin's vestibular glands. At the posterior edge of the vestibule is the fossa navicularis, while anteriorly, between the glans clitoridis and the urethral opening, is found the urethral sulcus. The urethral meatus opens on the urethral papilla. Anterolateral to the papilla can be seen the ostia of the paraurethral ducts leading from the periurethral glands.

The width of the introitus depends on the development of the vulva and the presence or absence of a hymen. Laterally at the edge of the introitus in multiparas are the carunculae hymenales (myrtiformes) that constitute the remains of the hymen.

The *clitoris* is formed of two crura that originate at the inferior pubic rami in the region of the interfascial perineal space (see p. 24). Both clitoral crura join to become the corpus clitoridis that ends in the rounded glans. The corpus consists of an ascending and a descending part. Between them is the angle at which the clitoris is joined to the symphysis pubis by means of the suspensory ligament (ligamentum suspensorium clitoridis). The crura are sometimes composed of a corpus cavernosum, although it is often attenuated and incompletely divided internally by a membrane, the septum of

---

Figure 2.

External female genitalia superimposed on skeletal structures, illustrating the clitoris and the vestibular bulb. *1* Glans clitoridis, *2* crura clitoridis, *3* bulbus vestibuli, *4* Bartholin's gland, *5* ischial tuberosity (palpable), *6* ischial spine, *7* perineal raphe, *8* tip of the coccyx (palpable).

See illustration on opposite page.

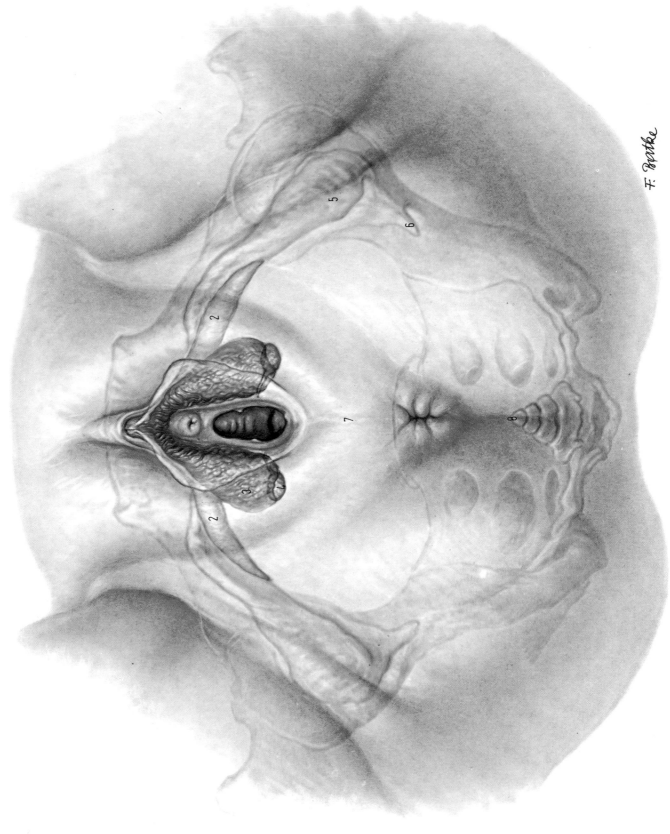

F. Brödke

Figure 2. *See legend on opposite page.*

the corpus cavernosum. The surface of this corpus cavernosum is composed of a tight, inelastic tunica albuginea. Additionally, the crura clitoridis are covered by the ischiocavernosus muscles that originate on the ischial tuberosity.

At the base of the labia majora lie the vascular *vestibular bulbs* (Fig. 2). They are situated very close to the urogenital diaphragm. Their posterior ends are distended, whereas they become thinner toward the symphysis. They are interconnected between the clitoris and the urethra. The two corpora cavernosa are covered by the bulbocavernosus muscles (musculus bulbospongiosus, musculus constrictor vaginae) that originate from the perineal body. These muscles radiate in contiguity with the ischiocavernosus muscles into the fascia that invests the body of the clitoris. The bulbocavernosus muscle is a relatively flat muscle covering both the vestibular bulb and Bartholin's gland. Its weakly constrictive components are strengthened by the levator sling.

The two pea-sized *Bartholin's glands* (glandula vestibularis major) (Fig. 2) contain mucous glandular elements and lie behind the deep transverse perineal muscles (musculus transversus perinei profundus). In part they are covered superficially by the thickened posterior ends of the vestibular bulbs. Each gland complex has a duct of about 2 cm. length that flows laterally from the vaginal introitus into the vestibule.

The *blood supply* of the external genital organs derives from both the internal and the external pudendal arteries. The pudendal artery, which originates from the femoral artery in the saphenous hiatus (or fossa ovalis), supplies the anterior labial arteries. These vessels in turn reach the anterior part of the labia majora. The posterior labial arteries arise from the internal pudendal artery, usually within Alcock's canal (see p. 22). They supply the posterior portion of the labia minora and majora.

The clitoris is supplied with blood by the deep clitoral artery (leading to the crura) and by the dorsal clitoral artery (to the glans). The latter is the terminal branch of the internal pudendal artery. The vestibular bulb gets its blood from the internal pudendal artery bilaterally via the vestibular bulbar arteries.

Blood drainage from the labia proceeds by way of the anterior and the posterior labial veins to both the internal and the external pudendal veins. The unpaired subfascial dorsal clitoral vein and the paired deep clitoral veins as well as the subcutaneous dorsal clitoral veins all originate from the clitoris. These veins are closely related to the pudendovesical plexus en route to the internal pudendal vein into which they can also flow by a more direct pathway. Moreover, some of the blood from the vestibular bulb enters the pudendovesical plexus. Another portion is expedited directly by way of the vestibular bulbar vein into the internal pudendal vein.

Lymph drainage from the external genitalia occurs through several lymphatic collecting channels to the superficial inguinal lymph nodes. Lymphatics from the corpus cavernosum travel along the internal pudendal vein to the interiliac node groups.

The *innervation* of the skin of the posterior aspects of the external genitalia (Fig. 3) consists of the posterior labial nerves that are branches of the internal pudendal nerve. The terminal branch of the pudendal nerve, the dorsal clitoral nerve, serves the skin in the area of the clitoris. The ilioinguinal nerve coursing through the inguinal canal (see p. 69) extends to the anterior portion of the labia in conjunction with the anterior labial nerve. The genital branch of the genitofemoral nerve also participates in the innervation of the external genitalia.

The anatomy of this area is particularly relevant, as it applies to surgical procedures involving the Schuchardt incision (see p. 80) and the operative treatment of Bartholin's gland cysts (see p. 608).

Figure 3.

Sensory innervation of the vulva: *yellow,* ilioinguinal nerve and genital branch of the genitofemoral nerve; *blue,* branches of the pudendal nerve.

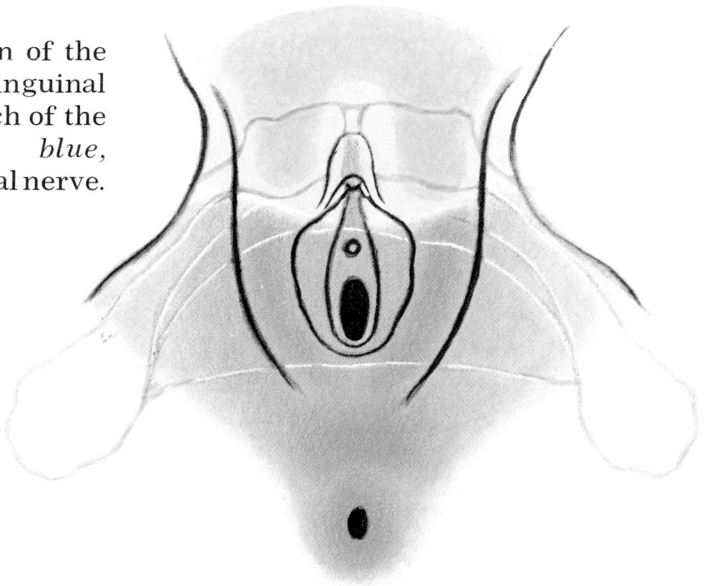

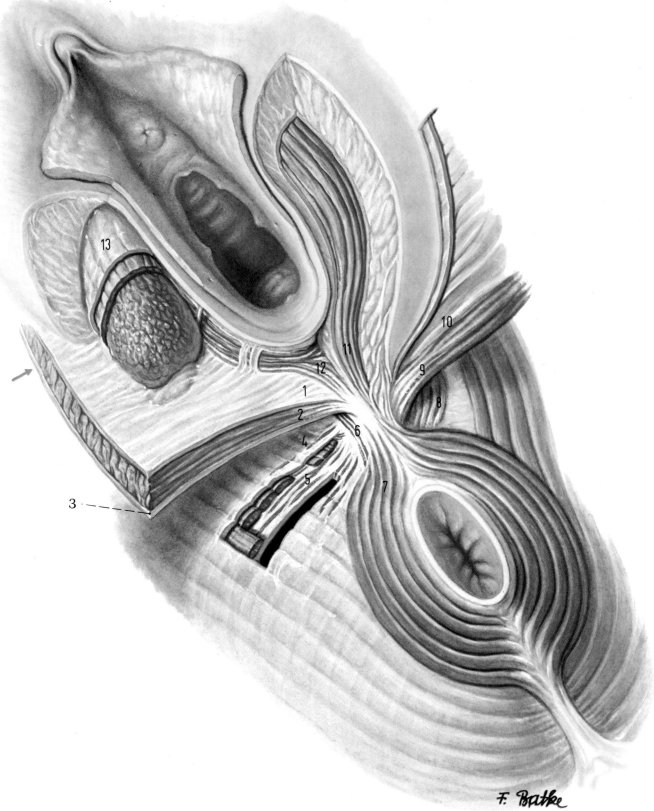

Figure 4.

Architecture of the perineum: *brown*, diagonally striated musculature; *red*, smooth muscle; *blue*, connective tissue; *yellow*, adipose tissue.

PERINEUM

The perineum (Fig. 1), situated between the vulva and the anus, is about 2.5 cm. long. Laterally toward the upper thigh, the perineum is bordered by the genitofemoral sulcus. The perineal raphe is a midline structure sometimes manifest as a skin fold that stretches between the pudendal aperture and the anus. The perineal body (*centrum tendineum perinei*) is the foundation of the perineum (Figs. 4 and 4a). The concept that it is composed entirely of connective tissue is actually incorrect because both smooth muscle and striated muscle bundles radiate into the coarse connective tissue that it contains.

In addition to the prerectal fibers of the levator ani muscle and smooth muscle fibers of the levator vaginae muscle, muscle bundles reach the perineal body from the deep and superficial transverse perineal muscles and the superficial portion of the external sphincter ani (Fig. 5) as well. Likewise, the medial muscle fibers of the deep transverse perineal muscle that form the urethrovaginal muscle (musculus sphincter vaginae), also enter it.

The bulbocavernosus muscle originates on either side of the perineal body. Some smooth muscle bundles stretch from the longitudinal muscle fibers of the rectum to the posterior wall of the vagina, participating as a rectovaginal muscle in the formation of

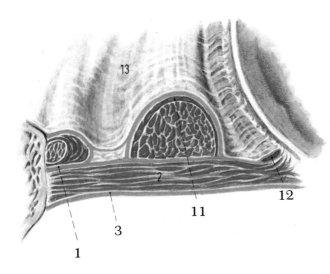

Figure 4a.

Section through the urogenital diaphragm (see arrow). *1* Inferior urogenital fascia, *2* deep transverse perineal muscle, *3* superior urogenital fascia, *4* inferior fascia of the pelvic diaphragm with smooth muscle fibers, *5* superior fascia of the pelvic diaphragm with smooth muscle fibers, *6* rectovaginal muscle, *7* external anal sphincter muscle, *8* prerectal fibers of the levator ani muscle, *9* superficial transverse perineal muscle, *10* deep transverse perineal muscle, *11* bulbocavernosus muscle, *12* urethrovaginal muscle, *13* perineal fascia (superficial).

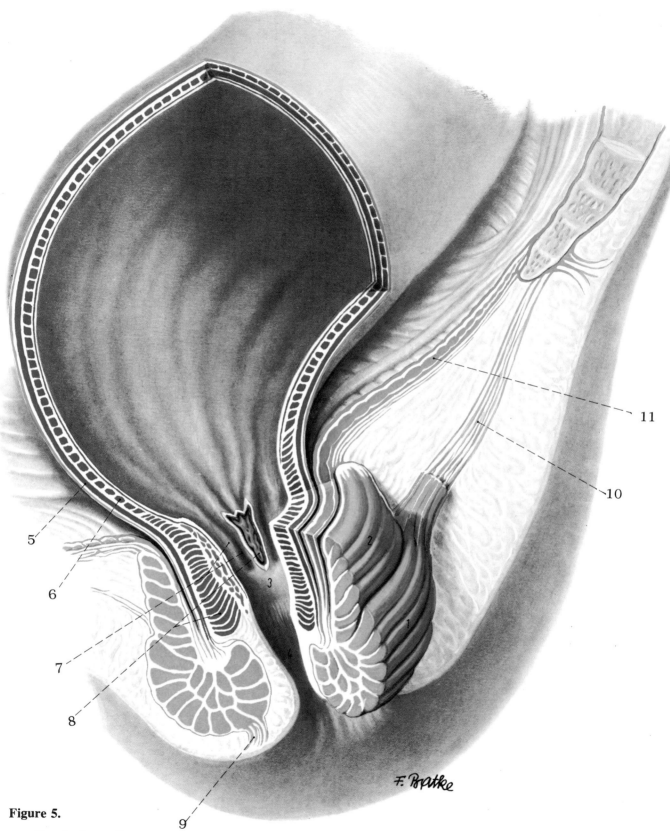

Figure 5.

    Semischematic representation of the anus and the external anal sphincter muscle. *1* Pars superficialis of the external sphincter, *2* pars profunda of the external sphincter, *3* zona intermedia, *4* zona cutanea, *5* longitudinal musculature of the rectum, *6* annular muscle of the rectum, *7* anal column and anal sinus, *8* internal anal sphincter muscle and venous plexus in an anal column, *9* pars subcutanea of the external anal sphincter, *10* anococcygeal ligament, *11* levator ani muscle and its fascia.

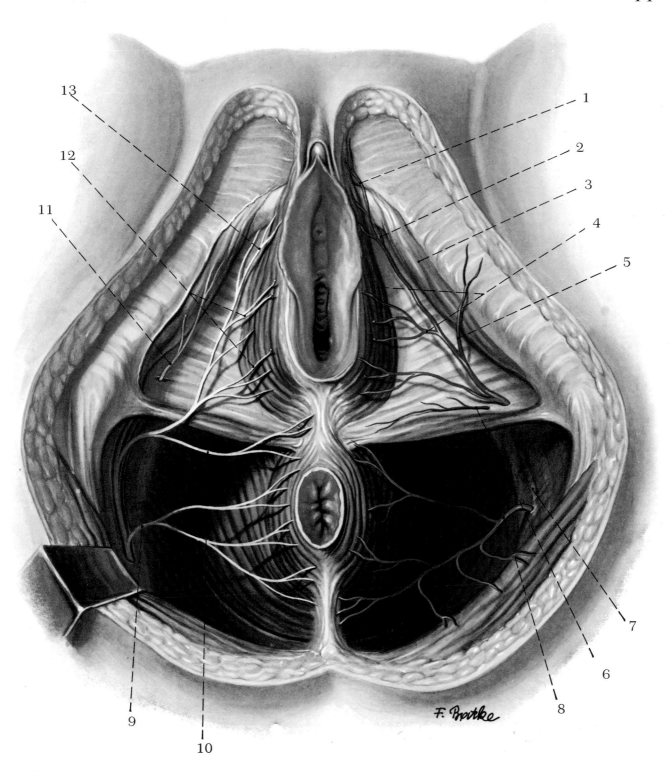

Figure 6.

The arteries and nerves of the pelvic floor as seen from below, demonstrating the branching of the internal pudendal artery and of the pudendal nerve. *1* Dorsal clitoral artery, *2* deep clitoral artery, *3* ischiocavernosus muscle, *4* bulbocavernosus muscle and the artery of the vestibular bulb, *5* posterior labial artery, *6* perineal artery, *7* internal pudendal artery in Alcock's canal, *8* inferior rectal artery, *9* anal nerve, *10* perineal nerve, *11* branch innervating the ischiocavernosus muscle, *12* posterior labial nerves, *13* dorsal clitoral nerve.

the perineal body. Smooth muscle fibers of the rectococcygeus muscle that are connected to the levator fascia are similarly attached. In addition to the muscle fibers arising from the inferior levator fascia (fascia diaphragmatis pelvis inferior, see p. 22), muscle bundles reach the centrum tendineum from the superior levator fascia (fascia diaphragmatis pelvis superior, see p. 22) as well as from both the superior and inferior fascias of the urogenital diaphragm (see p. 19). Finally, the connective tissue membranes that form the base of the labia majora and the superficial perineal fascia take part in the construction of the perineal body.

The centrum tendineum perinei thus appears as a large connective tissue structure permeated with a multitude of muscle fibers. All the elements listed, however, become nonfunctional if the perineum is destroyed and has to be restored by mass suturing that incorporates the levator pillar (see also p. 19).

The *blood supply* (Fig. 6) of the perineum is derived from the internal pudendal artery. It takes its origin at the internal pudendal artery, piercing through the foramen infrapiriforme and coursing around the ischial spine to reach the lateral wall of the ischiorectal fossa (see p. 22) by way of the small ischial foramen, where it enters Alcock's canal. There it gives rise to one or more perineal arteries. Veins with similar names accompany each of these arteries to handle the return of blood from the perineum.

Lymph drains from the perineum to the superficial inguinal nodes and thence to the lymph glands of the deep inguinal tract. The skin of the perineum is innervated by one or more nerves (Fig. 6) that are branches of the pudendal nerves. The pathways of these nerves follow the comparably named arteries.

The anatomy of the perineum is important with regard to colpoperineoplastic procedures (see p. 366), episiotomies (see p. 516) and repair of perineal lacerations (see p. 531).

Figure 7.

Projection of the bony pelvis and of the pelvic viscus on the external surface: *blue,* urinary tract, including ureters, urinary bladder and urethra; *red,* uterus and vagina; *black,* rectum.

See illustration on opposite page.

ANUS AND ANORECTAL CANAL

The anal orifice is situated in the gluteal cleft (crena ani) and borders the perineum posteriorly. Laterally, the anus is encroached on by levator fibers as well as by the external anal sphincter (musculus sphincter ani externus) into which the puborectal fibers of the levator ani muscle (see p. 18) radiate. The anus and the pars perinealis of the anal canal are fixed anteriorly by the perineal body and posteriorly by means of the anococcygeal ligament (Fig. 8).

The anus constitutes the opening of the anal canal (pars perinealis) and shows all transitions in its structure from the rectal wall to the skin. We shall detail this area only insofar as it is deemed necessary for those operative procedures to be discussed in this book.

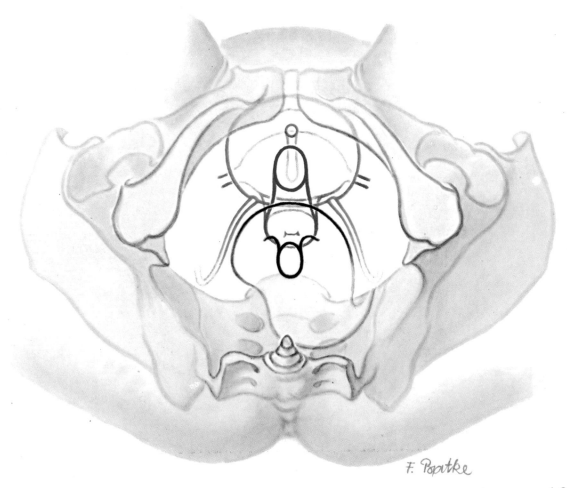

F. Popatke

Figure 7. *See legend on opposite page.* 13

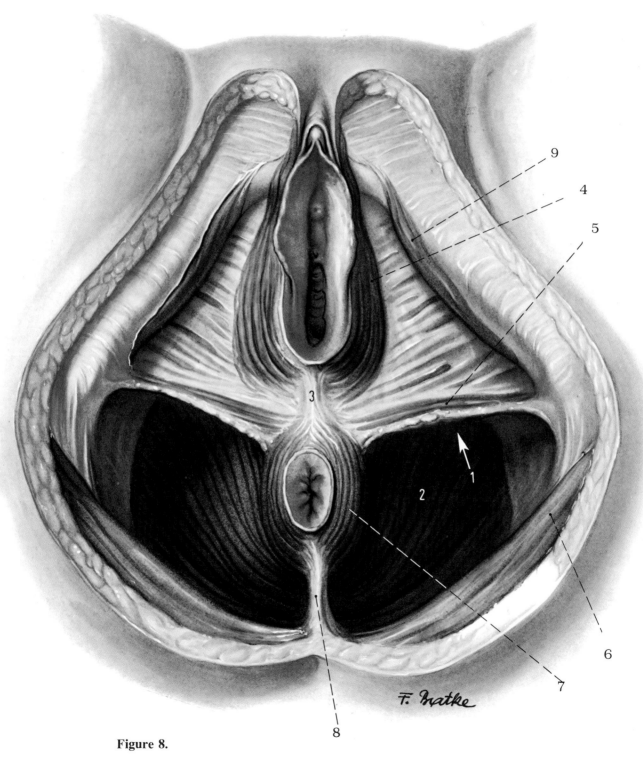

Figure 8.

Pelvic floor as seen from below with the urogenital diaphragm and the pelvic diaphragm in situ. *1* ischiorectal fossa (arrow), *2* levator ani muscle, *3* perineum, *4* bulbocavernosus muscle, *5* superficial transverse perineal muscle, *6* edge of the gluteus maximus muscle, *7* external anal sphincter muscle, *8* anococcygeal ligament, *9* ischiocavernosus muscle.

The anal canal begins with 6–10 anal columns that form longitudinal folds (zona hemorrhoidalis) and are supplied by venous plexuses. Outwardly, they are shut off by the anal valves. Between them are the niche-shaped cavities of the anal sinuses. Nonkeratinized squamous epithelium covers the anal columns, but cylindrical epithelium can be found overlying the intervening sinuses. This is an intermediate transitional zone that reaches up to the anocutaneous line. At this point the nonkeratinized squamous epithelium becomes cornified (cutaneous zone). The intestinal smooth muscle, which becomes intensified in the area of the zona intermedia, here abuts the internal anal sphincter muscle. A few bundles from this muscle section reach the coccyx as the rectococcygeus muscles.

The zona intermedia is also designated the *linea pectinata* and is of interest to the surgeon from various points of view. Besides the epithelial interface, there is a borderline of innervation. Moreover, a "watershed" exists here for lymph drainage, with collecting lymphatics leading to the superficial inguinal lymph nodes (see p. 73).

The skin in the anal region is thickened and invested with fatty tissue as well as circumanal and sebaceous glands. The anus is invested with the external anal sphincter where it passes through the pelvic diaphragm. Three sections of the sphincter can be distinguished (Fig. 5): a superficial portion, the pars subcutanea, radiates around the anus in the corium, while the pars superficialis surrounds the anus from the centrum tendineum to the anococcygeal ligament; the innermost layer, the pars profundum, rings the anus over a breadth of 3–4 cm.

The blood supply of the rectum flows by way of the inferior rectal artery (Fig. 6) that leaves Alcock's canal where it originates from the internal pudendal artery to penetrate the obturator fascia. Anastomoses with the medial rectal artery (which arises from the internal iliac artery) and the superior rectal artery (derived from the inferior mesenteric artery) guarantee adequate circulation even if the inferior rectal artery is interrupted. Drainage of blood occurs via veins bearing similar names that course in parallel with their corresponding arteries. A dense venous network in the hemorrhoidal zone represents the interconnection between inferior rectal, medial rectal and superior rectal veins. The superior rectal vein also provides a communication to the portal system.

Lymph drains to the superficial inguinal nodes as well as along the inferior rectal veins to the internal iliac lymph nodes. Lymphatic pathways also carry lymph to the sacral and rectal lymph glands. The skin in the anal region is innervated by the anal nerve branches of the pudendal nerves (Figs. 3 and 6). Knowledge of this region is important in the procedures involving repair of third degree perineal lacerations (see p. 531).

PELVIS

The bony pelvis is composed of the two innominate bones (os coxae) together with the sacrum and the coccyx. We shall deal here with the pelvic bones only as they are relevant to the operative procedures under discussion. It is necessary to distinguish between the true and the false pelves. They are separated by the linea terminalis that runs from the pubic bone over the linea arcuata to the sacral promontory. The true pelvis and its contents are of special interest.

Both innominate bones are attached anteriorly by the symphysis and posteriorly to the sacrum by means of the sacroiliac joint. Additionally, the sacrum is connected to the innominate bone bilaterally by way of the sacrotuberous and sacrospinous ligaments (Fig. 9). Check ligaments of lesser importance are the anterior interosseous and posterior sacroiliac ligaments. These three ligamentous groups lie near the sacroiliac joint.

The false pelvis is formed principally by the two ilia and is completed anteriorly in a band-like projection from the anterior superior iliac spine and the pubic tubercle through the inguinal ligament. Two portals to the upper thigh are formed between this band and the space formed by the iliac and pubic bones, subdivided by the iliopectineal line. These portals are the lacuna musculorum laterally and the lacuna vasorum medially (see p. 76).

The true pelvis is surrounded by bony structures on all sides. The obturator foramina can be found at the anterior lower wall of the pelvis. Anteriorly in the pelvic outlet, the pubic bone is palpable through the skin; posteriorly, one can palpate the ischial tuberosities and ischial spines as well. With the patient in lithotomy position, the ischial tuberosity is felt at the level of the perineum laterally at a distance of about 5–6 cm.

The sacrospinous ligament stretches between the sacrum and

Figure 9.

Representation of the ligaments of the pelvis and of the urogenital and pelvic diaphragms. *1* Sacrospinous ligament, *2* sacrotuberous ligament, *3* arcus tendineus of the obturator fascia (levator ani muscle), *4* obturator internus muscle (cross section) and the arcus tendineus fasciae obturatoriae, *5* inguinal ligament, arcus iliopectineus, *6* lacunar ligament, *7* transverse perineal ligament, *8* obturator membrane. *a* Deep transverse perineal muscle, *b* urethrovaginal muscle, *c* prerectal fibers, *d* puborectal muscle, *e* pubococcygeus muscle, *f* iliococcygeus muscle, *g* coccygeus muscle. *See illustration on opposite page.*

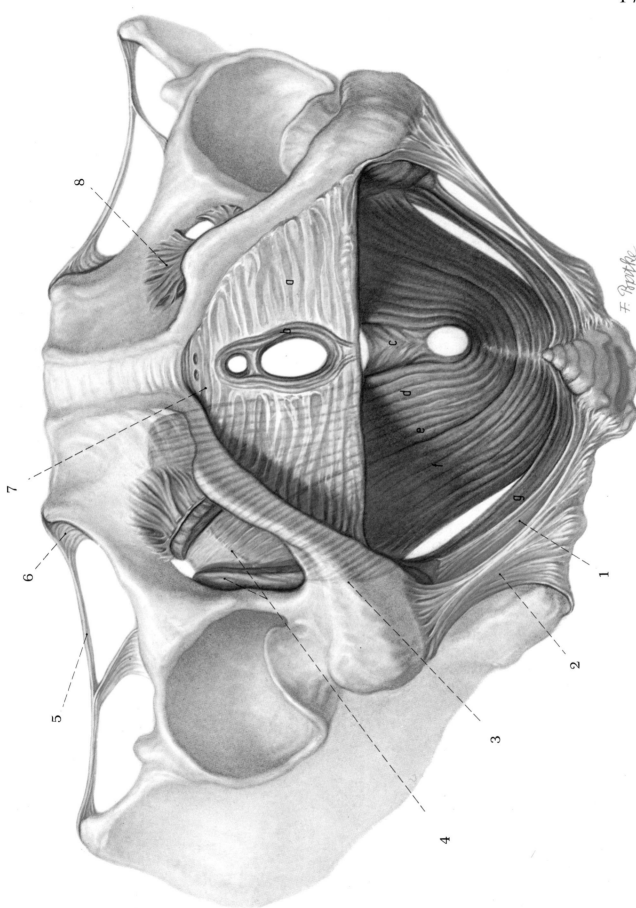

Figure 9. *See legend on opposite page.*

the ischial spine and forms the minor ischial foramen (Fig. 9) in conjunction with the sacrotuberous ligament that is attached to the ischial tuberosity. In a more superior location is the larger or major ischial foramen, bordered by the incisura ischiadica major and subdivided into a suprapiriform and an infrapiriform foramen by the musculus piriformis. The bony aspects of the smaller foramen ischiadicum minus, which lies more caudally, are formed by the incisura ischiadica minor. The internal pudendal vessels and the pudendal nerve wind under and around the ischial spine to reach Alcock's canal (see p. 22) in the wall of the ischiorectal fossa.

The true pelvis contains the following organs: urinary bladder, urethra and ureters, vagina, uterus and adnexa, as well as the rectum (Fig. 7).

Musculature and Fascia

The osseous wall of the true pelvis is invested muscularly by the piriform and internal obturator muscles. The musculus piriformis originates at the anterior surface of the second to the fourth sacral vertebrae laterally to the sacral foramina. It exits from the true pelvis by way of the foramen ischiadicum majus and reaches the greater trochanter. The internal obturator muscle takes its origin at the bony edge of the obturator foramen and from the obturator membrane. It courses through the small ischial foramen, using the incisura ischiadica minor as a buttress to insert into the greater trochanter as well. At its origin, it averts the obturator canal located at the upper edge of the obturator foramen.

The obturator vessels and nerve exit from the true pelvis via the obturator canal. Alongside the obturator canal are four openings in the sidewall of the true pelvis that serve as passages for vessels and nerves, including (1) the suprapiriform foramen for the superior gluteal vessels and nerve, (2) the infrapiriform foramen for the inferior gluteal vessels, the inferior gluteal nerve, ischial and posterior femoral cutaneous nerves, the internal pudendal vessels and the pudendal nerve, and finally (3) the small ischial foramen (foramen ischiadicum minus) for the internal pudendal vessels, the pudendal nerve and the obturator internus muscle. Additionally, lymph vessels course through all of these foramina.

PELVIC FLOOR

Muscular Foundation

The pelvic floor is formed by two fibromuscular layers, the pelvic diaphragm and the urogenital diaphragm. Neither alone closes the pelvis completely, but closure is functionally effective, nevertheless, because the superimposed layers are arranged so that the open portions are not aligned.

The funnel-shaped *pelvic diaphragm* (Figs. 6, 8 and 9) consists of the *levator ani muscle* and the coccygeus muscle. The levator ani takes its origin at the pubic bone near the symphysis and reaches over the arcus tendineus of the obturator fascia (arcus tendineus musculus levatoris ani) to the ischial spine. The three segments of the levator ani muscle are discernible bilaterally, corresponding to the course of its muscle fibers. The puborectalis muscle encompasses mainly those fibers that form the so-called levator pillar, laterally intertwining with the external anal sphincter muscle on the one hand, and posteriorly, forming a sling for contralateral traction of the rectum on the other. The prerectal fibers course toward the perineum in association with the puborectalis muscle to form the levator pillar. Together with the perineal body (see p. 9) they border the levator portal, the urogenital hiatus, beginning at the anal hiatus. Smooth muscle fibers radiate alongside these striated muscles from the levator to the perineal body looping around the vagina in the form of the musculus levator vaginae.

The remaining levator fibers comprise the pubococcygeus and the iliococcygeus muscles that reach the tip of the coccyx by way of the rectococcygeus aponeurosis in conjunction with the smooth muscle bundles of the rectococcygeus. Parts of the pubococcygeus and puborectalis muscles radiate into the vaginal wall as the pubovaginalis muscle.

The levator portal is very important insofar as it is impossible to avert intestinal descensus if the levator pillar is pulled apart (Figs. 10 and 11). During construction of an artificial perineum (see p. 382), one must take care with the puborectalis muscle, because both sides have to be drawn together (Figs. 12 and 13) in order to ensure a secure pelvic floor to support the bowel.

The pelvic diaphragm is completed posteriorly by the coccygeus muscle that courses from the ischial spine to the coccyx and sacrum. As a rule the pelvic diaphragm is innervated by a long branch from the sacral plexus.

The *urogenital diaphragm* is of particular importance here because it provides needed support for the levator portal, which is naturally larger in women. The urogenital diaphragm is mainly formed by the deep transverse perineal muscle that terminates in the perineal wedge. The diaphragm, permeated with connective tissue, originates from the lower ischium and the inferior ramus of the pubis and courses to the urogenital hiatus that it encircles to yield a urogenital sphincter (musculus urethrovaginalis, musculus sphincter vaginae). Anteriorly, its muscular layer changes into the transverse perineal ligament (ligamentum transversum perinei, ligamentum praeurethrale), which forms the anterior part of the

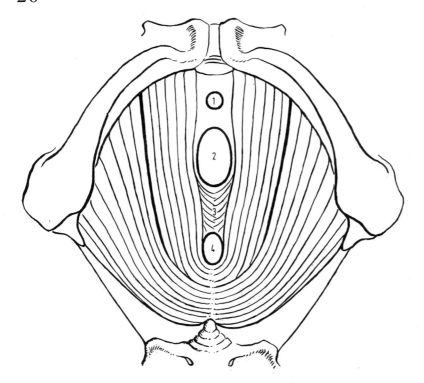

Figure 10.

Schematic presentation of the pelvic diaphragm (levator ani muscle) showing a normal large levator portal as seen from below. *1* Urethra, *2* vagina, *3* prerectal levator fibers, *4* anus.

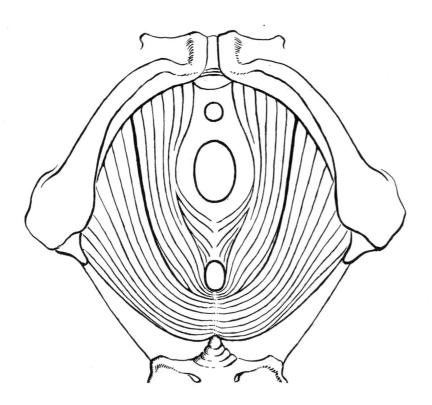

Figure 11.

The pelvic diaphragm (levator ani muscle) shown schematically with an enlarged levator portal viewed from the perineum.

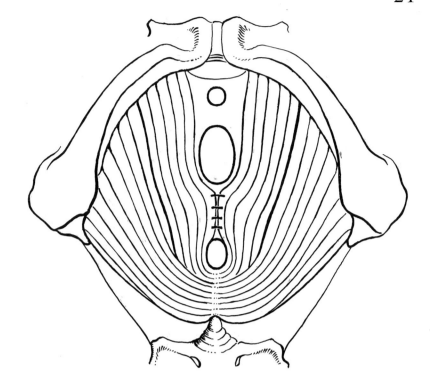

Figure 12.

Artificial construction of perineum accomplished by suturing both levator pillars between the vagina and the anus, seen from below.

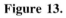

Figure 13.

The reconstructed perineum becomes further strengthened by suturing both bulbocavernosus muscles together between the vagina and the anus, viewed from below.

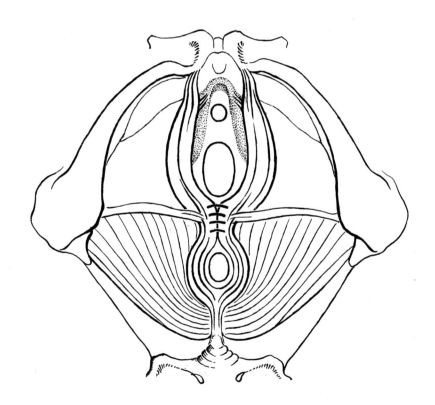

urogenital diaphragm in conjunction with the ligamentum arcuatum pubis. The free edge of the diaphragm is strengthened by the superficial transverse perineal muscle that arises from the ischial tuberosity and inserts into the perineal body.

The urogenital diaphragm is innervated by branches of the pudendal nerve. The bulbocavernosus and ischiocavernosus muscles are located superficially on the urogenital diaphragm (see p. 4).

The anatomy of this region is important in radical vaginal operations (see p. 80), colpoperineoplasties (see p. 366), procedures for vaginal atresia (see p. 392), repairs of perineal laceration (see p. 531) and constructions of artificial vaginae (see p. 650).

Fascial Base

The muscular pelvic diaphragm is covered by a fascia on both its superior and inferior surfaces. The superior fascia (fascia diaphragmatis pelvis superior) extends from the arcus tendineus of the obturator fascia (arcus tendineus musculus levatoris ani) to reach the lateral pelvic fascia (obturator fascia, fascia pelvis parietalis). Posteriorly, it attaches over the sacrum as well as with that portion of the fascia located above the piriform muscle. The inferior fascia (fascia diaphragmatis pelvis inferior) proceeds to the levator pillars. Both superior and inferior levator fascias, as derivatives of the pelvic parietal fascia, are connected to the fascias of the rectum, vagina and urethra, all portions of the pelvic visceral fascia.

Because the pelvic and the urogenital diaphragms are arranged in strata, the inferior fascia of the pelvic diaphragm also passes over the superior fascia of the urogenital diaphragm. The superior urogenital fascia proceeds anteriorly under the transverse perineal ligament (ligamentum praeurethrale) and posteriorly on the free edge of the urogenital diaphragm to the inferior urogenital fascia. Near the levator muscles, the fascias of the pelvic diaphragm fuse with those of the urogenital diaphragm so that the hiatus urogenitalis between them is closed. The ischiorectal fossa is formed posterolaterally where the pelvic parietal fascia approaches the lateral pelvic sidewall. The pelvic parietal fascia in this area corresponds to the subdiaphragmatic portion of the obturator fascia. It possesses a duplication (sometimes designated as fascia lunata) that creates an interfascial canal (Alcock's canal, canalis pudendalis) between its

Figure 14.

Schematic demonstration of the layers of the anterior vaginal wall: *yellow,* vaginal mucosa; *pink,* vaginal muscularis; *blue,* vaginal fascia (the muscle layer of the bladder can be seen through a window in the fascia vaginalis): *orange,* mucosa and muscle of the vagina (both layers are separated together as the vaginal wall).

See illustration on opposite page.

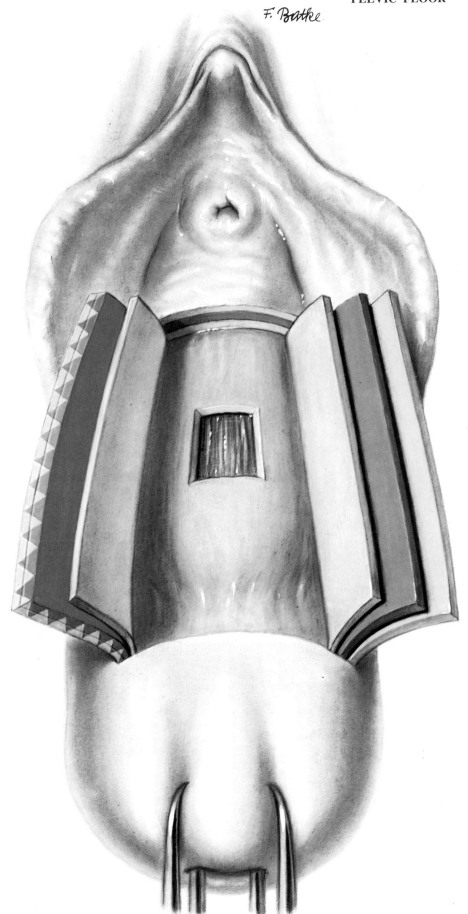

Figure 14. *See legend on opposite page.*

two leaves to accommodate the internal pudendal vessels and pudendal nerve.

Closer to the skin than the inferior fascia of the urogenital diaphragm (or the deep perineal fascia) lies the *perineal fascia* (fascia perinealis, Colles fascia, fascia perinei superficialis), which is fused with the inferior urogenital fascia at its posterior edge. Thus, an interfascial space, the spatium interfasciale perinei, is formed between the arcus pubis and the posterior edge of the urogenital diaphragm. The nomenclature applied to the fascias in the literature differs widely so that disparate descriptions of individual layers are often found. The superficial perineal fascia proceeds into the superficial connective tissue membranes (Camper's fascia) of the pubic area on the one hand, and into those of the thigh on the other (see p. 71).

PELVIC CONTENTS

The true pelvis (Fig. 7) contains the vagina, the uterus and the adnexal structures, including the uterine tubes and the ovaries, all constituents of the internal female genital apparatus, as well as the pelvic portions of the ureters, the urinary bladder, the urethra and the rectum. These structures are connected with each other and with the parietal wall by means of a connective tissue membrane that has special significance as a pelvic support and as a pathway to guide the course of vessels and nerves.

VAGINA

In its relaxed, undistended state the vagina is flattened anteroposteriorly from the introitus to the posterior fornix. Because the portio vaginalis (see p. 29) of the uterus inserts into the upper vagina, the vaginal vault is formed around the portio of the vaginal fornix. The posterior wall is longer (about 11 cm.) than the relatively shorter overlying anterior wall (about 8 cm). The fornix forms an ir-

---

Figure 15.

Schematic representation of the layers of the posterior vaginal wall. *Yellow,* mucosa of posterior vagina; *pink,* musculature; *blue,* fascia vaginalis in situ, fascia rectalis (including the rectal musculature); *orange,* posterior vaginal mucosa and muscularis as conjointly dissected.

See illustration on opposite page.

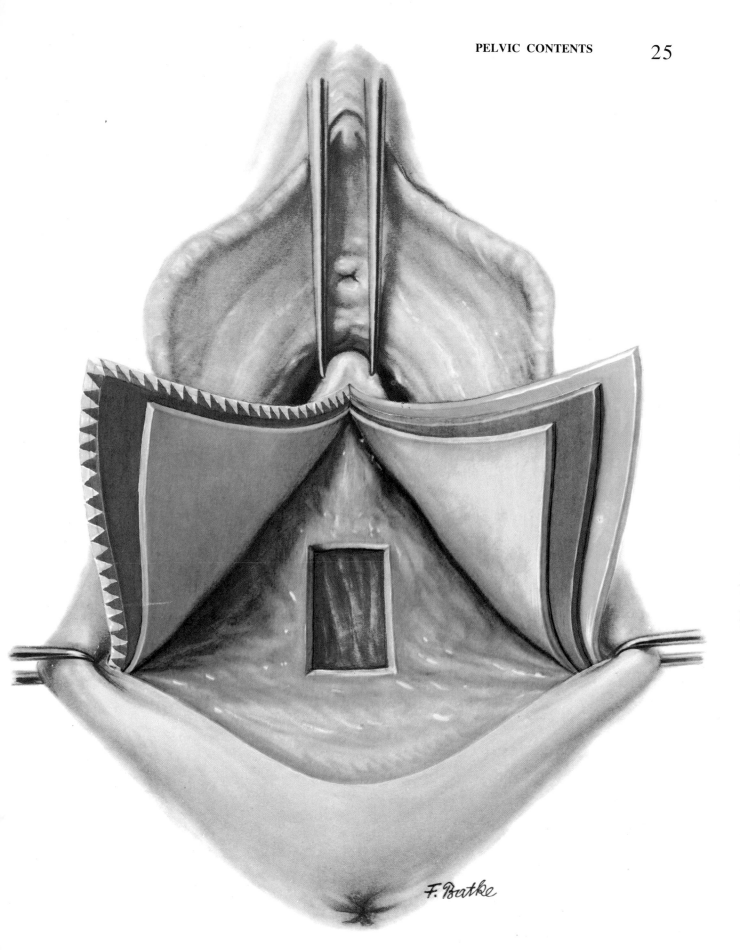

Figure 15. *See legend on opposite page.*

regularly deep groove that circles the portio and characteristically protrudes more deeply into the posterior fornix and more shallowly into the two lateral fornices and the anterior fornix.

Layers of the Wall

The wall of the vagina consists of a tunica mucosa, a tunica muscularis and a tunica adventitia, called the fascia vaginalis. In surgical dissection of the vaginal wall the mucosal and muscular strata are usually represented as a common layer separate from the vaginal fascia (Figs. 14 and 15). Care must be taken to ensure that the fascia vaginalis maintains a close relationship with the bladder fascia (fascia vesicalis, see p. 50).

The greyish-red mucosa is covered by a squamous epithelium that ordinarily does not undergo cornification, but can keratinize in association with prolapse. The lamina propria contains much elastic tissue as well as a lattice work of collagen fibers. Diagonal folds, the rugae vaginales, are seen in the undistended mucosa of the adult vagina. These form the anterior and posterior columna rugarum on the respective longitudinal vaginal wall borders. The anterior border is bounded by a band of vertical muscle fibers from the tunica muscularis. This muscular layer is in intimate relationship with the mucosa, and, as already mentioned, tends to be surgically dissected in conjunction with the mucosa. There is no tunica submucosa in the vagina. In the distal continuation of the columna rugarum anterior, there is a slight forward arch, the carina urethralis, contained by the close relationship between vagina and urethra.

The mucosa is subject to menstrual cyclic changes in that it is thicker and looser during the secretory phase and premenstrually than in the proliferative or postmenstrual phases. The mucus part of the vaginal secretions does not arise in the few isolated glands found in the upper vagina (and which participate in the cyclic changes that the cervical glands undergo), but rather from glands in the endocervical canal.

The tunica muscularis comprises smooth musculature and a network of elastic fibers. The muscle fibers are in a fencelike arrangement in rhomboid shapes such that the vertical axis of the rhombus is perpendicular to the vertical axis of the vagina. The muscle is thicker in the anterior wall where many muscle fibers bend vertically to form the foundation of the columna rugarum anterior. There are numerous vascular plexuses within the muscle layer. These plexuses are, in turn, well developed in the region of the posterior rugal columns, here resembling the corpus cavernosum. The muscularis in the upper vagina is only loosely connected with the tunica adventitia (fascia vaginalis) in contrast to the close interrelationship near the introitus. Here there is also intimate connective tissue connection between the fascia vaginalis and the fascias of neighboring organs, designated rectovaginal and urethrovaginal septa, respectively (Fig. 16).

In the posterior fornix, the fascia vaginalis is missing and a portion of vagina is covered by peritoneum for a distance of 1–2 cm. This constitutes the shortest distance from the posterior vaginal vault to the peritoneal cavity via the culdesac of Douglas (excavatio rectouterina).

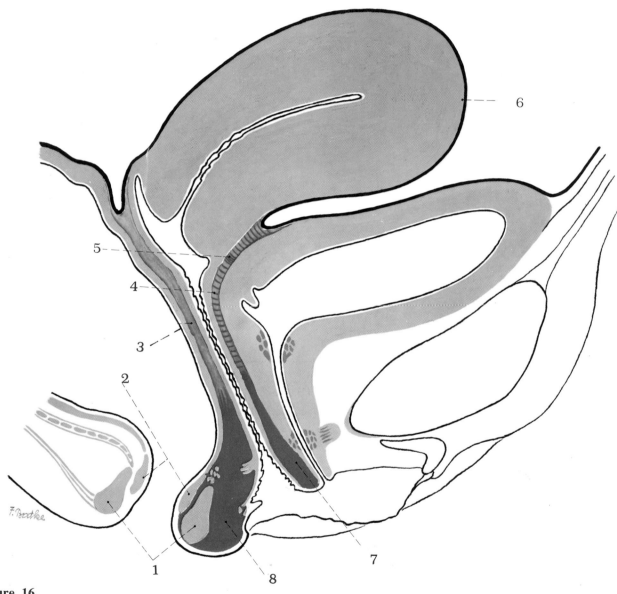

Figure 16.

Midline diagrammatic section of the perivaginal connective tissue. *1* External anal sphincter muscle, *2* internal sphincter, *3* loose areolar connective tissue between vaginal and rectal fascias in the rectovaginal space, *4* areolar connective tissue between vaginal and vesical or urethral fascias in the vesicovaginal or urethrovaginal spaces, *5* supravaginal septum, *6* peritoneum, *7* dense connective tissue completely occupying the urethrovaginal space, *8* dense fibrous tissue filling the rectovaginal space.

Relationship to Adjacent Organs

As already stated, a close relationship exists at the anterior wall near the introitus to the urethra through the *urethrovaginal septum.* In the upper vagina, the anterior wall is loosely connected to the base of the bladder, whereas laterally, the two ureters approach the vagina. Dorsally, in the posterior fornix, the vagina closely juxtaposes the peritoneal cavity and the rectum. More distally, there are connective tissue fibers that form a relationship near the introitus in the *rectovaginal septum* analogous to that seen anteriorly.

Laterally, the vagina is surrounded by fibers of deep transverse perineal muscle (see p. 19) in the form of the sphincter urogenitalis. A few of its muscle bundles can encircle the vagina and the urethra as a sphincter urethrovaginalis (musculus urethrovaginalis, musculus sphincter vaginae, see p. 19). In the intact pelvic diaphragm, the levator pillars can be felt laterally through the vagina. A few fibers of pubococcygeus and puborectalis muscles radiate as the pubovaginal muscle into the vaginal wall. These fibers are sometimes called musculus constrictor (or compressor) vaginae. The bundle of connective tissue that runs from the vagina to the lateral pelvic wall and contains blood vessels, lymphatics and nerves can be considered collectively as the *paracolpium.*

Vaginal Blood Supply and Lymphatics

The vaginal artery, a branch of the uterine artery, and smaller branches of the inferior vesical artery, the inferior rectal artery (Figs. 26 and 27) and the internal pudendal artery reach the vagina laterally by way of the paracolpium to supply it with blood. Sometimes these branches anastomose at the posterior wall of the vagina, a form of vertical anastomotic network, an arterium azygos vaginae.

Vascular drainage occurs bilaterally to the internal iliac veins via the uterovaginal plexus that is located in the paracolpium and the parametrium. There are anastomotic connections with the internal pudendal vein and with the veins of the external genitalia as well.

Lymph is drained (Fig. 20) from the upper half of the vagina by way of the lymphatics that also serve to collect lymph from the cervix uteri through the cardinal ligament to reach the interiliac nodes. A few lymph vessels, after crossing the ureter near its confluence with the bladder, also reach the interiliac lymph nodes, especially those located most caudally. From the lower vagina, the lymph vessels (a) accompany the vaginal artery laterally to the ureter to terminate in the interiliac nodes also. Other lymphatics course through the paravesical space (see p. 64) to the inferior gluteal nodes. Additional lymphatics reach the superior gluteal nodes in coassociation with the vaginal artery. Finally, the afferent lymphatics of the lower vagina

(b) also drain into inguinal lymph nodes.* A few lymph vessels from the posterior vaginal wall (c) reach the rectal nodes by way of the rectovaginal septum.

Innervation

Near the introitus, the vagina is supplied by sensory branches of the pudendal nerve, while the remaining sensory and autonomic fibers originate in Frankenhäuser's plexus (plexus pelvinus Frankenhäuser), reaching the vaginal wall in association with arterial branches. Knowledge of this region is a prerequisite for all vaginal operations.

UTERUS

The pear-shaped uterus has an anterior surface (facies vesicalis), a posterior surface (facies rectalis) and laterally rounded aspects (margines laterales). It consists of the corpus and the cervix (collum). The latter can be distinguished by a slight constriction at the isthmus uteri. The uppermost portion of the corpus (above the mouths of the uterine tubes) is called the fundus uteri. The cervix is divisible into a portio supravaginalis (occupying two thirds of the structure) and a portio vaginalis (one third). In older women, the portio vaginalis becomes flattened and foreshortened. The portio is that portion of the uterus that is admitted into the vagina, bearing the external os (orificium uteri externum) at the distal extremity between its anterior and posterior lips. The orifice represents the external opening of the cervical canal. The other end of the canal enters into the flattened, triangular endometrial cavity. The uterine tubes open into the upper lateral corners of the cavity. The internal os is the site of the junction of the cervical canal and the endometrium.

Physiologically, the uterus is in a median axial position, anteverted (with the vertical axis of the uterus perpendicular to the axis of the vagina) and anteflexed (with a forward inclination of the corpus with regard to the cervix).

Architecture of the Uterine Wall

The uterus consists of three layers: (1) its mucosa, the endometrium, (2) its muscle layer, the myometrium, and (3) a serosal layer, the perimetrium, which covers it almost completely. There is no serosal perimetrium in the anterior aspect of the cervix.

---

*Strictly speaking, lower vaginal lymphatic channels have not been demonstrated to drain directly into the regional nodes in the femoral triangle. They do, however, anastomose with lymph vessels that arise in the vestibule to reach these glands secondarily. — Ed.

The reddish *endometrium* at rest is approximately 1 mm. thick; it is covered with cylindrical epithelium and forms fine folds in the cervical canal on both anterior and posterior walls. Periodically, these little folds transform into one median vertical fold. They are called plicae palmatae by virtue of their palm-like appearance. Inside the endometrial cavity, the mucosal surface is flat and softer than that in the area of the cervix. The lamina propria is relatively thick, firm and immovably fixed to the myometrium. Within the lamina propria in the corpus region are the uterine glands, whereas, in the lamina propria of the cervix, there are many blood vessels and cervical glands. The transition from the cervix to the corpus occurs in the isthmic canal. For further details on the mucosa, the reader is referred to the relevant publications on histology.

The *myometrium* consists of smooth musculature. It is in contiguity with the muscle of the uterine tube and, in the area of the cervix, with the vesicouterine and rectouterine muscle. Three layers can be distinguished on the basis of blood-vessel content. Muscle fibers radiate into the ligamentum latum (the broad ligament) from the superficial muscle layer.

The *serosa* (perimetrium) covers almost all the uterus except that it does not reach the cervix anteriorly. Laterally, the serosa becomes the two leaves of the ligamentum latum (plica lata). The shallow pouch of the excavatio vesicouterine is formed anteriorly while the deep excavatio rectouterina appears posteriorly as the culdesac of Douglas (see also p. 27).

Uterine Connective Tissue

The uterus possesses two lateral mesenteries or mesometria, the ligamenta lata uteri (or broad ligaments). At the free edge of the broad ligament is the round ligament (ligamentum teres uteri, ligamentum rotunda, chorda uteroinguinalis) that courses anteriorly toward the inguinal canal. The utero-ovarian ligament (ligamentum ovarii proprium, chorda utero-ovarica) travels from this site laterally toward the ovary. The fallopian tube is also found here with its mesentery, the mesosalpinx (Fig. 17).

The parametrial connective tissue is contiguous laterally with that of the paracolpium and is interspersed with blood and lymph vessels and nerves. Its fibrous components are loosely interwoven with smooth muscle fibers. At the lateral aspects of the upper pole of the cervix, the connective tissue becomes augmented and more compactly organized into the cardinal ligaments (ligamentum cardinal Kocks, ligamentum transversum colli Mackenrodt, retinaculum colli, lateral cervical ligament, see p. 61). They reach the upper fascia of the levator ani muscle close to the ischial spine. Lateral to the cervix two fibromuscular bands are found that pull the cervix forward toward the bladder as well as backward to the rectum. These are the vesico-uterine ligaments (or muscles) that represent the medial portion of the bladder pillar (see p. 63). They pass toward the bladder, approaching the lateral connective tissue of the bladder

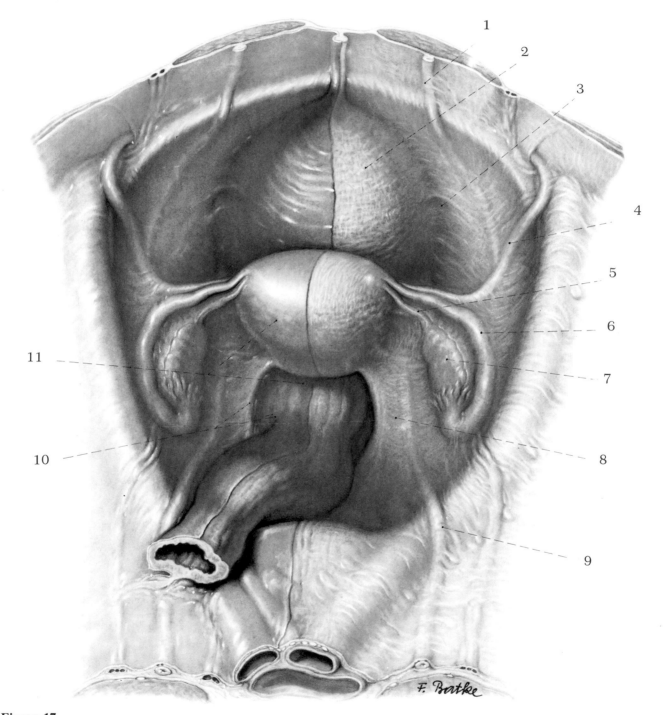

Figure 17.

View of the true pelvis from above with the peritoneum on the right side removed. *1*, Lateral umbilical plica with obliterated umbilical artery, *2* urinary bladder, *3* paracystium, *4* round ligament, *5* utero-ovarian ligament, *6* uterine tube, *7* ovary, *8* paraproctium, *9* ureter, *10* uterosacral plica and rectum, *11* excavatio rectouterina and uterus.

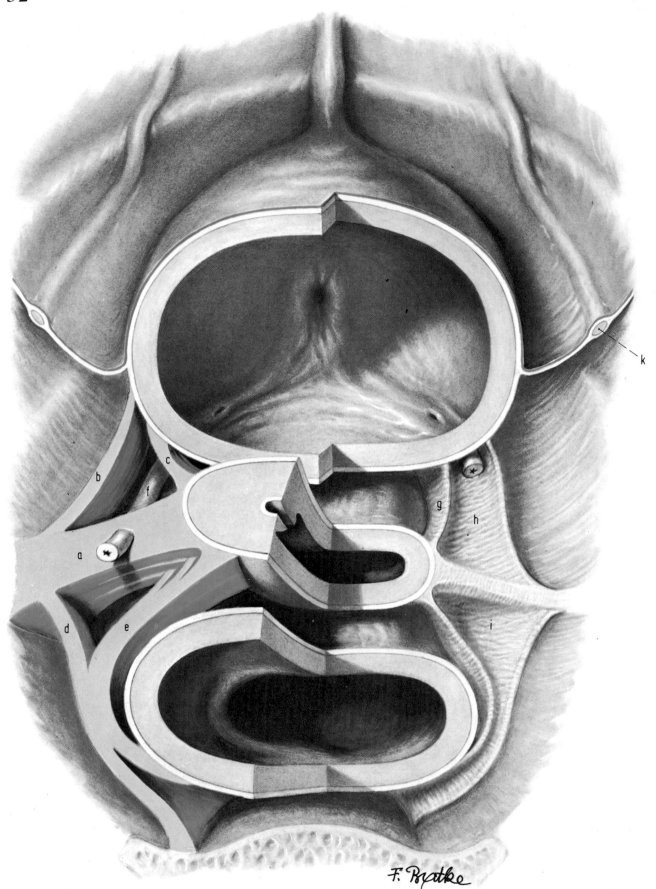

Figure 18.   *See legend on opposite page.*

(paracystium) in the region of the bladder base. The rectouterine ligaments follow the rectouterine plica at the lateral aspects of the cul-desac of Douglas, turning up on either side to reach the rectum. They constitute the medial components of the rectal crura (see p. 63), reaching to the rectal fascia, to the retrorectal connective tissue and to the sacrum at the level of the second to the fourth sacral vertebrae.

Among the three fibromuscular structures we have referred to here, the cardinal ligament has greatest practical importance and is a principal pathway for vessels and nerves. At its upper edge, it is crossed by the ureter. Anteriorly in the midportion is found another taut connective tissue bundle of importance to the gynecologist, the septum (or ligamentum) supravaginale (see Fig. 16) that courses from the posterior wall to the bladder.

Blood Supply

The uterine blood supply (Fig. 19, see also Figs. 26 and 27) comes by way of the uterine artery, a major branch of the internal iliac artery. It flows in the parametrium above the cardinal ligament, thereby crossing the ureters en route to the cervix. The ureteral crossing occurs about 2 cm. distally from the uterus. Adjacent to the cervix, the uterine artery turns upward and reaches the tubal angle in a tortuous coiling manner. There it separates into its terminal branches, a tubal and an ovarian ramus. It sends out short subserosal branches to the uterine wall along its route at the lateral margin of the uterus. These enter the anterior and posterior surfaces of the uterus and anastomose with those of the opposite side.

The uterine artery may give off a vaginal artery branch either before or after it crosses the ureter. Sometimes it can divide near the uterus into an ascending branch, which is a continuation of the main vessel, and a descending cervicovaginal ramus. Where it crosses the ureter, the uterine artery also gives rise to a ureteric branch (see pp. 39, 47). The end branches, the ovarian and tubal rami, anastomose with branches of the ovarian artery (which originates in the abdominal aorta) and transport blood to the uterine wall.

Veins also leave the uterus at its lateral margins and course

---

Figure 18.

Section through bladder, uterus, vagina and rectum with connective tissue pillars (somewhat schematized) shown in blue and peritoneal cut-edge in green. *a* Cardinal ligament, *b* lateral part of the bladder pillar (containing vessels and nerves), *c* medial part of the bladder pillar (the vesicouterine ligament sometimes containing a vesicovaginal artery), *d* lateral portion of the rectal pillar (with vessels and nerves), *e* medial part of the rectal pillar (uterosacral ligament), *f* ureter in the loose connective tissue (not shown) of the bladder pillar, *g* loose connective tissue between vagina and bladder, *h* areolar tissue in bladder pillar, *i* loose fibrous tissue in rectal pillar, and *k* umbilical artery.

See illustration on opposite page.

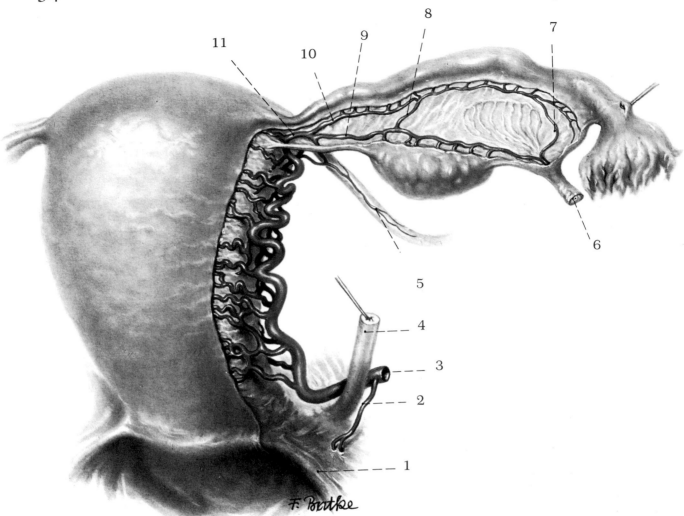

Figure 19.

Arteries of the uterus and the adnexa. *1* Uterosacral plica, *2* vaginal artery, *3* uterine artery, *4* ureter (raised up), *5* round ligament with its artery, *6* ovarian artery, *7* tubal branch of the ovarian artery, *8* anastomotic branch, *9* ovarian ramus of the uterine artery, *10* tubal ramus of the uterine artery, and *11* uterine artery.

through the broad ligament. They can be divided into three groups bilaterally, draining the fundus, the corpus and the cervix, respectively, and are interconnected to each other by anastomoses. The veins from the corpus and the cervix form the uterine venous plexus that envelops the uterine artery. Veins from the area of the fundus drain blood mainly via the ovarian veins to the inferior vena cava. The uterine venous plexus flows into the uterine veins, one of which proceeds cranially over the ureter, and the other caudally under the ureter. Blood from the cervical and vaginal veins flows from the vaginal venous plexus into the lower uterine veins. A rare pathway for drainage from the uterine fundus courses with the round ligament to the subcutaneous veins in the region of the external inguinal ring (see p. 67).

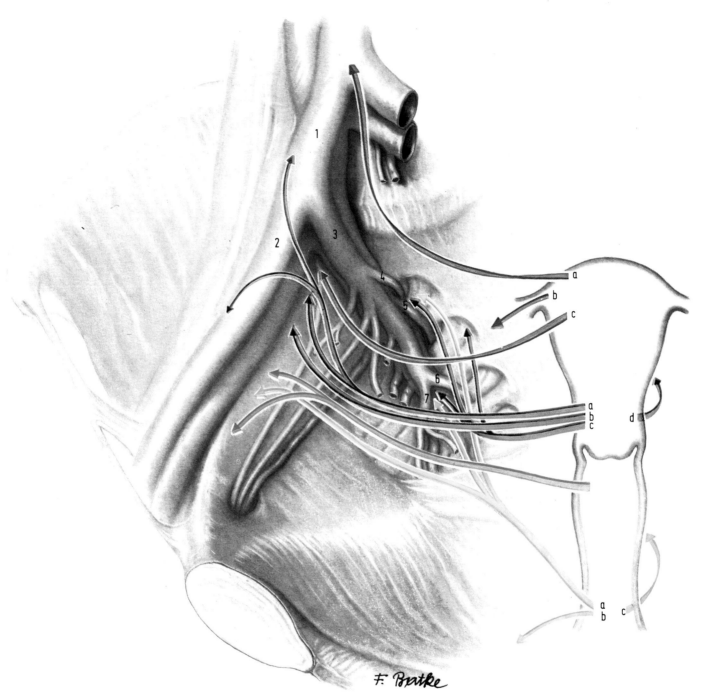

Figure 20.

Lymphatic drainage from the uterus and vagina, shown schematically. *Red*, lymph pathway from the fundus and corpus uteri; *blue*, from the cervix; *green*, from the upper portion of the vagina; *yellow*, from the lower vagina. *1* Common iliac artery, *2* external iliac artery, *3* internal iliac artery, *4* superior gluteal artery, *5* superior gluteal vein, *6* inferior gluteal artery, *7* internal pudendal artery. See text (pp. 28 and 34) for details of the specific pathways (here designated alphabetically) for each of the three drainage groupings.

ampulla and thence enters the uterus by way of the tubal isthmus and the pars intramuralis (pars uterina). The ostium uterinum opens into the endometrial cavity.

The salpinx is located in the upper free edge of the broad ligament between the round ligament and the utero-ovarian ligament. The tubal mesentery, the mesosalpinx, is short near the uterus with only about 3–4 cm. of potential elasticity in the relatively immobile isthmic portion. The ampullary part of the mesosalpinx is longer, about 7–8 cm., and bow-shaped so that this aspect of the tube is mobile. In the mesosalpinx are found smooth muscle fibers and occasionally the vestigial remnants of the urogenital anlage, the epoophoron. These rests may join to form a longitudinal duct, which runs parallel to the tube (made up of Wolffian ductile elements), and a transverse duct (derived from Wolffian body remnants). Less often, one can also see a pedunculated structure, the appendix vesiculosa, comprising residua from the Wolffian body.

Layers of the Wall

The tubal wall thickness narrows from the abdominal ostium (2 mm.) to the uterine ostium (0.5 mm.). The innermost layer, the tunica mucosa, forms many folds that disappear toward the uterus. The epithelial layer consists of ciliary, secretory and small peg cells. The cyclic development of all lining cells is dependent on the menstrual phases.

The tunica muscularis is attached to the mucosa without a submucosa and consists of an outer longitudinal and an inner annular muscle fiber layer. In the annular layer juxtaposed fibers run both transversely and circularly. A loose subserosal layer, containing vessels, separates the tunica muscularis from the serosa. The serosal epithelium abuts the luminal mucosa in the area of the fimbriae.

Relationships to Adjacent Organs

Bilaterally, the tube has several surfaces of contact with neighboring organs. Thus the anterior surface touches the posterior bladder when the bladder is distended. The right tube is in contact posteriorly with the rectum and in some circumstances with the vermiform appendix. As a consequence, where the appendix is particularly long, secondary adhesions can develop. The posterior surface of the left tube is in close relationship with the sigmoid and its mesentery.

Vessels and Nerves

Blood reaches the tube distally from the branches of the ovarian artery (see Fig. 19) and proximally by way of tubal anastomotic

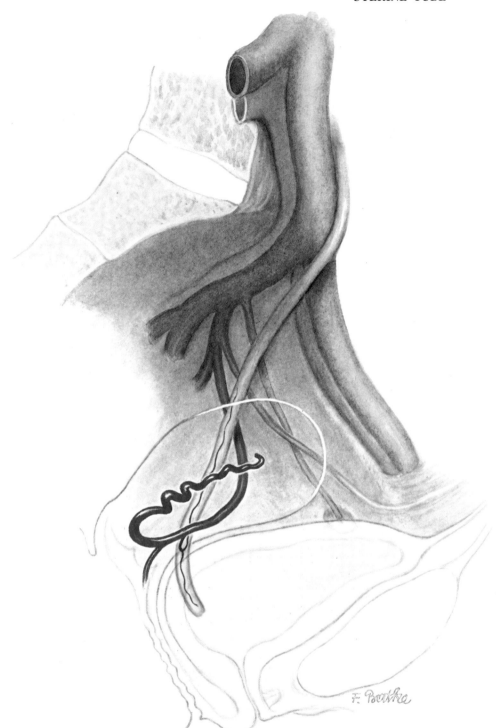

Figure 22.

Schematic section illustrating the course of the ureter and the uterine artery. A ureteral artery is given off from the uterine artery where it crosses the ureter. Medially, a cervicovaginal branch is sometimes encountered.

branches of the uterine artery. Drainage of blood occurs through comparably-named veins.

The subserous lymphatics of the isthmus interconnect with those of the corpus uteri, while lymph vessels stemming from the muscularis join those of the ovary (see p. 42). The innervation is derived from the ovarian plexus and the uterine plexus.

The anatomy of the uterine tube is significant in radical vaginal surgery (see p. 80), vaginal hysterectomy (see p. 214) and colpoceliotomy (see p. 591).

OVARY

In the adult female, the ovaries are situated bilaterally in the fossa ovarica (see Fig. 17), which is the peritoneal indentation cavity formed by the angle of the common iliac artery at its bifurcation. At the base of the fossa ovarica runs the obturator nerve; the ureter traverses its posterior edge.

The ovary of an adult woman may be as large as 5 cm. in length and up to 3 cm. wide and 2 cm. thick. The pole in contact with the tube, the tubal extremity, can be distinguished from the pole directed toward the uterus, the uterine extremity. The ovarian surface facing the uterus is the facies lateralis and the surface directed inward is the facies medialis. The dorsal edge is the margo liber, whereas that which borders the mesentery is called the margo mesovaricus. The mesovarium is a short mesentery which arises from the posterior surface of the broad ligament.

Superficially, the ovary is covered by the so-called "germinal" epithelium that becomes the peritoneal epithelium at the Farré-Waldeyer line at the margo mesovaricus. Immediately beneath the epithelium lies a tunica albuginea to which the ovarian stroma connects. The medullary portion must be distinguished from the cortical aspects. The connective tissue of the ovarian medulla blends into that of the mesentery at the hilus (which marks the beginning of the mesovarium). The vessels and nerves are also contained here. Relevant histological sources should be consulted regarding details of the surface covering and other fine structures of the ovary.

Figure 23.

View of the bladder base from below with the vaginal wall and the connective tissue (vaginal and vesical fascias) completely removed. Inset: *a* direction of the ureters in this area when the bladder is in normal position; *b* ureteral course in association with descensus uteri; *c* with uterine prolapse.

See illustration on opposite page.

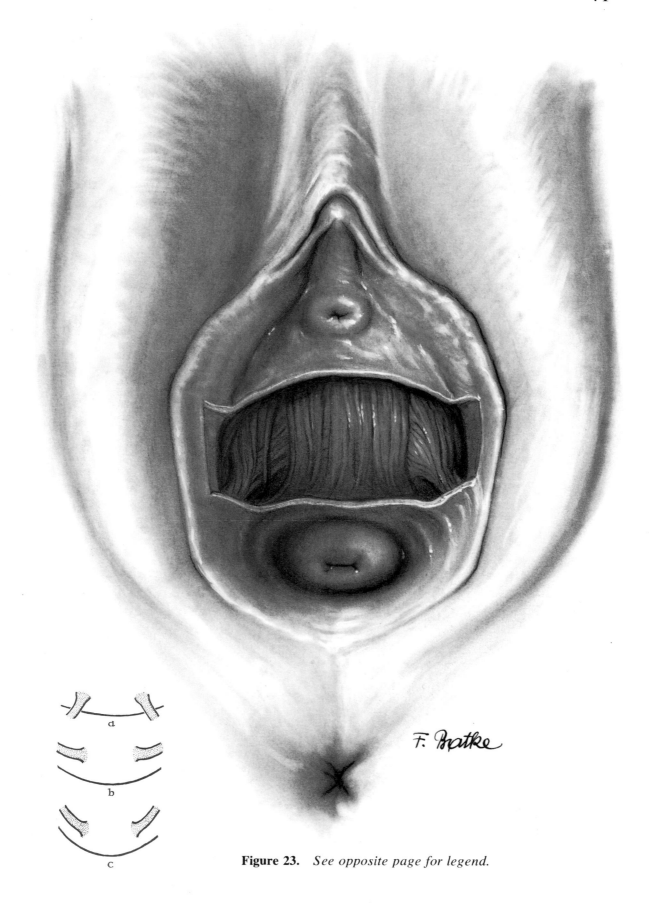

Figure 23. *See opposite page for legend.*

Ovarian Supports

The uterine tube lies above the ovary and is in direct contact by way of the fimbria ovarica. A peritoneal fold, containing connective tissue, runs from the tubal extremity of the ovary; this is the suspensory ligament of the ovary (ligamentum infundibulopelvicum, ligamentum suspensorium ovarii), which reaches to the lateral pelvic wall in the neighborhood of the external iliac vein. In addition to connective tissue, this structure contains the ovarian vessels, nerves and lymphatics. The utero-ovarian ligament (ligamentum ovarii proprium, chorda utero-ovarica) courses from the uterine extremity of the ovary as a thickened fold on the posterior surface of the broad ligament to reach the uterus where it disappears in the angle of the tube.

Vessels and Nerves

The blood supply (see Fig. 19) to the ovary on the distal side comes via the ovarian artery from the abdominal aorta through the infundibulopelvic ligament. On the proximal side, the ovarian anastomotic branch of the uterine artery reaches the ovary by way of the utero-ovarian ligament. Both arteries anastomose in the mesovarium and send out small branches into the ovary from this anastomosis. Blood drains from the ovary by like-named venous channels. In the hilar region, these veins form a plexus, the bulbus ovarii, which can distend with blood and even reach the size of the ovary.

Lymph drainage occurs by way of channels that course in the infundibulopelvic ligament along the ovarian vessels up to the aortic lymph nodes (node lymphatici aortici lumbales). Because they are interconnected with lymphatic efferents from the tube as well as with those from the uterine fundus, the possibility exists that lymph from the ovary follows a common pathway with lymph from the uterine fundus (see p. 34) to reach the corresponding lymph nodes.

The ovarian nervous plexus (derived from the aortic plexus) runs along the ovarian artery to the ovary. It contains both autonomic and sensory fibers supplying the ovarian surface. The importance of anatomical knowledge of the ovary is shown in radical vaginal operations (see p. 80).

Figure 24.

Position of the ureters and the bladder in uterine prolapse. The ascending ureter in its normal original state (black) becomes almost horizontal when the bladder sinks anteriorly (blue). In more extensive cases with moderate (green) or severe (pink) descensus uteri, the ureter descends vertically.

See illustration on opposite page.

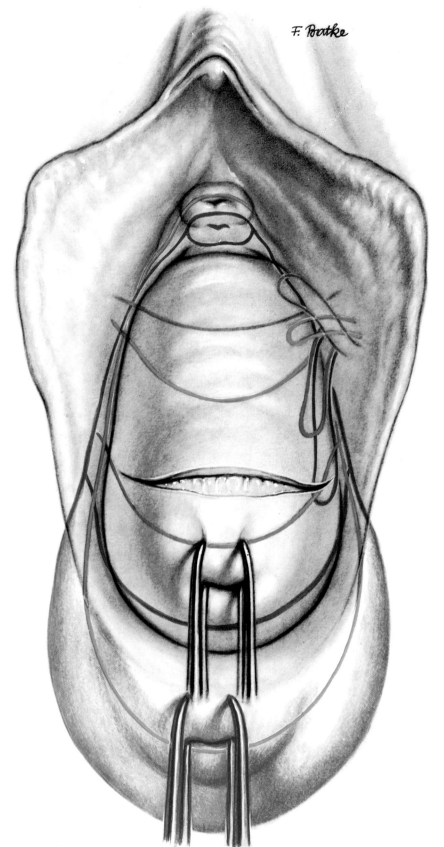

Figure 24. *See legend on opposite page.*

Figure 25.

Uterine prolapse with cystocele and rectocele in a median sagittal section. The peritoneal cut-edge is green. *1* Urinary bladder, *2* round ligament, *3* urethra, *4* cystocele, *5* excavatio vesicouterina, *6* external cervical os, *7* excavatio rectouterina, *8* rectocele, *9* rectum, *10* uterine tube and ovary.

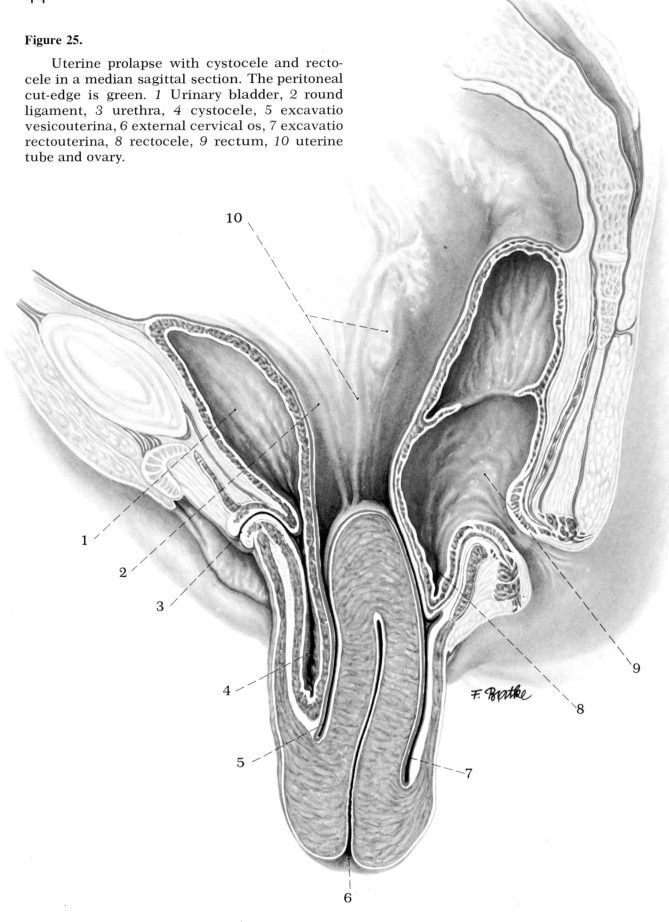

F. Boptke

PELVIC URETER

The pelvic portion of the ureter, about 15 cm. long (Fig. 22), extends from the linea terminalis to the bladder. In practical terms one can distinguish three parts of the pelvic ureter. First, a descending portion describes a curve that is convex outwardly, changing into the ascending retrovesical part at the so-called "ureteral knee." The ascending segment, together with the intramural part, enters transversely into the bladder wall and opens into the bladder cavity at the ureteral orifice.

Layers of the Wall

The wall of the ureter is three-layered. The innermost layer, the tunica mucosa, is formed into folds during contractions (so that the lumen forms a star-shape) and carries a transitional epithelium. There is no submucosa so that the tunica muscularis, consisting of a loose inner longitudinal muscle layer and a dense outer circular layer, connects directly with the mucosa. In the anterior part of the

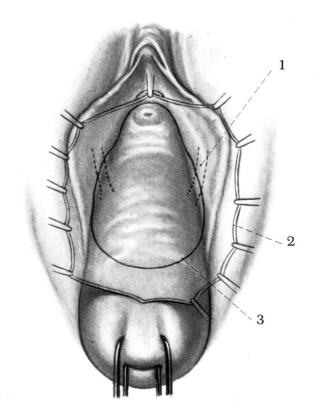

Figure 25a.

Schematic view of the operative field in prolapse of the bladder and the vagina, showing section of the ureter near the bladder, the cut-edge of the vaginal wall and the operative margins diagrammatically. *1* Ureteral course near the bladder, *2* separated vaginal wall, *3* edge of operative field.

intramural segment, longitudinal fasciculi of fibers are also present outside the circular muscle layer. In the region of the intramural portion, the ureteral musculature changes into the bladder musculature (Figs. 23, 28 and 28a). The outermost layer is a connective tissue covering, the tunica adventitia, which contains the blood vessels that supply the ureter. This adventitia can enter into a closer, more intimate relationship with the surrounding connective tissue.

Relationships to Adjacent Organs (Figs. 17, 22, 31 and 32)

On entering the true pelvis, the ureter crosses the common iliac artery near its bifurcation. Sometimes it lies somewhat more laterally and instead crosses the external iliac artery. The crossing point corresponds to the approximate location of the sacroiliac articulation. The ureter describes a descending outward convex bow in the first part of the pelvic portion. Laterally lie the ovarian vessels; anteriorly, it reaches the base of the infundibulopelvic ligament. Further down, it is situated medially to the internal iliac artery (hypogastric artery) and its branches, as well as medially to the obturator nerve, reaching the posterior border of the fossa ovarica subperitoneally behind the ovary. Subsequently, the ureter loses its close relationship to the peritoneum and courses through the cardinal ligament above the rectal pillar. Before it reaches the rectal pillar (and even afterwards), the ureter possesses a connective tissue sheath, originating from its adventitia (ureteral lamina) that is connected to the rectal pillar. Presupposing normal locations of the pelvic viscera, the ureter describes a convex descending curve here, then ascends through the bladder pillar to the base of the bladder. This transition in the ascending portion, as aforementioned, is described as the ureteral knee (Figs. 23 and 24).

In its passage through the cardinal ligament, the ureter is crossed by the uterine artery (Figs. 22, 26 and 27) and lies about 1.5–2 cm. from the cervix. However, in isolated cases it can be as close as 1 cm. to the cervix or as far as 4 cm. distant from it. Before the ureter reaches the base of the bladder, it is still in close contact with the anterior vaginal fornix.

The ascending portion of the ureter can alter its direction as a consequence of a change in the position of the genital organs (Fig. 23). Thus, in the case of a cystocele, for example, the ureter approaches the bladder laterally only; when the cystocele is associated with uterine prolapse, the ureter also descends toward the bladder (Fig. 24).

Vessels and Nerves

The pelvic ureter receives its blood supply (Figs. 26 and 27) from several different arteries and a certain degree of variability is expected. In addition to a branch of the ovarian artery that reaches the ureter, this structure receives blood by way of the rami from common iliac, internal iliac, iliolumbar, superior gluteal and medial rectal arteries. All of these supplying vessels are very variable in their number and caliber as well as in their antecedent arterial sources.

The ureteral portion near the bladder is of particular interest to the gynecologist because damage to all supplying vessels at this site can lead to inadequate tissue perfusion and thence necrosis of this section. This diminished perfusion occurs even though the very delicate adventitial arterial network possesses numerous anastomoses; in a healthy ureter these anastomoses are insufficient to provide adequate blood supply alone. Damage to the adventitia during ureteral curettage may also interrupt the blood supply here and cause necrosis.

In the part of the ureter near the bladder, we encounter a branch of the uterine artery that arises from the uterine artery where it crosses the ureter. Usually, this vessel separates into an ascending and a descending ramus; the descending branch anastomoses with branches from the superior and inferior vesical arteries to supply the ureter. Additionally, a branch of the vaginal artery also frequently leads into the adventitial network. Because of the numerous supplying arteries, any one of the branches, including the vessel from the uterine artery, can be ligated during the Schauta operation with impunity. It must be stressed, however, that the ureteral adventitia and its blood supply must be preserved intact (see above).

The vesical plexus drains blood from the pelvic ureter via the uterine plexus directly to the internal iliac vein and the ovarian vein. Lymphatics follow the blood vessels to reach the internal iliac and common iliac nodes.

The innervation of the pelvic portion of the ureter comes by way of the pelvic plexus as well as the vesical plexus. In addition to autonomic fibers, sensory nerves also reach the ureter via the important vesicourethral ganglion located near the entrance of the ureter into the bladder. The anatomy of the pelvic ureter is important for all vaginal operations.

URINARY BLADDER

The bladder (Fig. 17) lies above and behind the symphysis in the space of Retzius (spatium praeperitoneale). At its lower surface in the area of the bladder base (fundus vesicae), it is connected with the urogenital diaphragm. The vesical fundus continues anteriorly in an upward direction in front of the corpus uteri, rising to the bladder vertex (vertex vesicae). At the inner surface of the bladder base is the trigone (trigonum vesicae) with posterior angles formed by the ureteral ostia (orificia ureterica). Between the ureters that

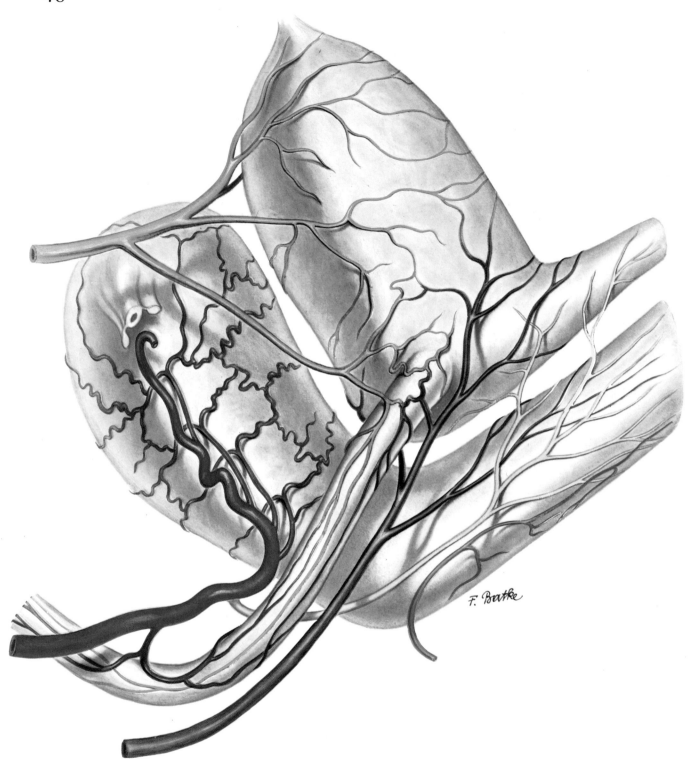

Figure 26.

Blood supply of the portion of the ureter near the bladder, of the uterus in this area, of the more central parts of the urethra and of the vagina, as seen from the side. *Red*, uterine artery; *yellow*, vaginal artery; *blue*, superior vesical artery; *violet*, inferior vesical artery; *green*, branch of the inferior rectal artery.

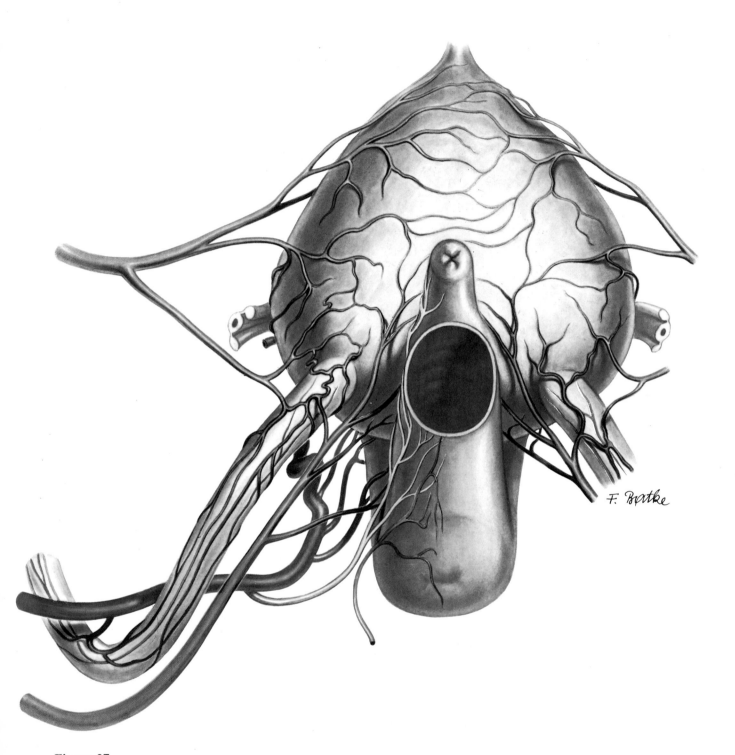

Figure 27.

Anteroinferior view of ureteral, uterine and urethral blood supply, color-coded as in Figure 26.

empty here, stretches the plica interureterica. Anteriorly, the bladder trigone is bordered by the urethral orifice whose lumen forms a half-moon in the closed state by virtue of a projection of the mucous membrane.

Layers of the Wall

The reddish tunica mucosa possesses a transitional epithelium and a loose lamina propria, which is rich in blood vessels. Except in the trigone, there is an adjoining submucosa. The immovable mucosa of the trigone is directly juxtaposed to the subjacent tunica muscularis (see Fig. 28). A definite layer of muscularis cannot be found here, but it appears more as a netlike reticular arrangement of muscle fibers. Only in isolated areas, e.g., the dorsal part, is there a three-layered architecture with outer longitudinal fibers (musculus detrusor vesicae), middle annular and spiral fibers (musculus compressor vesicae) and an inner reticular layer.

In the region of the trigone, the musculature is distinguished by its fine muscle bundles and its content of elastic fibers. From there, muscle fibers of the outer layer reach the anterior pelvic wall at the symphysis in the form of the pubovesical muscle (ligamentum pubovesicale), and additionally as the vesicouterine muscles within the vesicouterine ligaments to reach the uterus. Posteriorly, a diagonal muscle enlargement is formed; the ureteral musculature continues into this structure to yield the structural base for the plica interureterica. Longitudinal muscle fibers course directly beneath the mucosa, converging toward the urethral ostium that they surround from behind like a bridle. In this way, a half sphincter is formed. From the anterior aspect, a corresponding reversed half sphincter forms around the opening made in the annular fibers, and functions to close the urethral orifice. Additionally, a smooth muscle lissosphincter urethrae (Hayek) converges towards the urethra.

The outer layer of the bladder is partially formed of serosa, partly by a tunica adventitia (fascia vesicalis). The posterior bladder wall is covered by peritoneum, that is only loosely adherent to the muscularis. When the bladder is empty, one or more transverse plicae course diagonally across the posterior wall of the bladder in the form of reserve peritoneal folds. The fascia vesicalis is firmly attached to the fascia vaginalis in places and is especially in intimate connection with the fascial adventitia of the cervix in the supravaginal septum (ligamentum supravaginale) as shown in Figure 16.

Attachments of the Bladder (Figs. 16, 31, 32, and 33)

The base of the bladder lies approximately at the level of the lower edge of the symphysis pubis to which it is densely adherent by

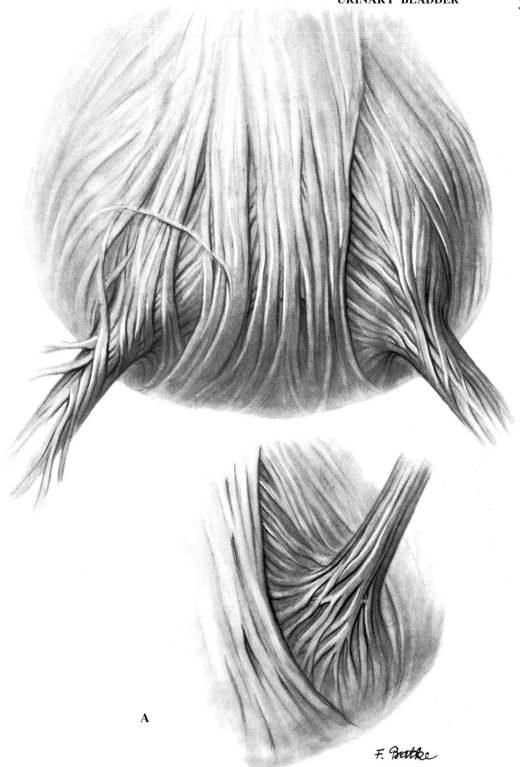

A

F. Bratke

Figure 28.

The musculature of the fundus of the urinary bladder, seen from below. The ureteral muscle radiates into the deep layer of the bladder muscle.

Figure 28A.

Ureterovesical junction shown with the ureter retracted upward.

means of the fascia of the superior urogenital diaphragm. The bladder is anchored anteriorly over the pubovesical ligament in the area of the symphysis. The bladder base is also in relationship to the vagina where loose areolar connective tissue is found between the vesical fascia and the vaginal fascia. This structure is termed the vesicovaginal septum by various authors. In actuality this undoubtedly is not a real septum but rather consists merely of connective tissue that can be condensed during the course of a surgical operation to evoke the impression that it is a septum or a ligament. It is more correct to speak here of a vesicovaginal space that is filled with loose connective tissue and is situated between the fascial layers. It is only between the cervix and the bladder that one encounters a true condensation of connective tissue that can be described as the supravaginal septum (see Fig. 16).

Laterally to the bladder is the loose areolar tissue of the paracystium that also possesses denser fibers as well. The latter are arranged to form the bladder pillars that course from the anterior part of the cardinal ligament to the bladder base. The medial part of the bladder pillar originates near the cervix. It corresponds to the vesicouterine ligament (or vesicouterine muscle by virtue of its smooth muscle content) and sometimes contains a vesicovaginal branch from the uterine artery. The lateral portions, through which course most of the blood vessels, are designated in the American literature as the "lateral ligaments."*

A wider band courses from the vertex of the bladder; this is the median umbilical ligament (ligamentum vesicoumbilicale, ligamentum umbilicale medianum) that contains the obliterated urachus reaching to the umbilicus.

Vessels and Nerves

The blood supply (Figs. 26 and 27) comes by way of a pair of vesical arteries. The superior vesical artery (often consisting of two branches) originates at the beginning of the umbilical artery and terminates in the upper lateral part of the bladder pillar. The inferior vesical artery, a direct branch of the internal iliac artery, reaches the bladder by passing through the lower lateral aspect of the bladder pillar. Numerous anastomoses exist between these two vessels. Moreover, the bladder may be supplied by branches arising from the uterine and the vaginal arteries.

Like-named veins form a plexus within the bladder pillar. This plexus represents a portion of the vesical plexus and is connected to

---

*More fully designated the lateral ligaments of the bladder, these fibroareolar condensations course from the sides of the bladder into the pelvic fascia. Because they contain smooth muscle components, they are often also referred to as rectovesical muscles. — Ed.

both the uterine and vaginal venous plexuses near the cardinal ligament. The anterior vesical veins course from the anterior surface of the bladder; they unite into a single trunk to join the pudendal plexus or the dorsal clitoral vein. By way of these tributaries, blood can drain not only to the internal iliac veins but also to the femoral veins.

The lymphatic efferent vessels reach from the bladder pillars to the interiliac nodes. Innervation occurs by way of the vesical nerves from the vesical plexus, which is formed in turn from the pelvic plexus. The pelvic plexus derives its parasympathetic elements from the sacral cord (nervi splanchnici pelvini) and its sympathetic fibers from the lumbar portion of the spinal cord (plexus hypogastricus superior). The major part of the vesical nerves innervates the lateral aspect of the bladder pillar, laterally to the vesicouterine ligament. These nerves may therefore be damaged during the division of the bladder pillars and in the operative preparation of the paravesical space.

It is essential to be familiar with the anatomy of the bladder during radical vaginal surgery (see p. 80), vaginal hysterectomy (see p. 214), anterior colporrhaphy (see p. 330), Manchester procedure (see p. 462) and the operative treatment of vesicovaginal fistula (see p. 666).

URETHRA

The relatively short (3–5 cm.) female urethra extends from the bladder through the levator portal to empty into the vaginal vestibule at the external urethral ostium. For purposes of expediency, the gynecologist should distinguish between two parts of the urethra: (1) the upper portion, loosely attached to the vaginal fascia, called the pars superior (or pars libera), and (2) the contrasting pars inferior (or pars fixa) that is bound down by the urethrovaginal septum.

Layers of the Wall

The tunica mucosa exhibits a very variable epithelial layer, consisting of transitional or cuboidal epithelium or even of a squamous covering. Glands can be found in the lamina propria; their numbers increase toward the external urethral orifice. A submucosa separates the mucosa from the tunica muscularis. The latter consists of smooth muscle with superimposed layers of diagonally striated muscle. The smooth muscle is composed of an inner longitudinal and an outer annular fiber layer. Both layers are essentially continuations of the bladder musculature. The fiber bundles of the pubovesical muscle run from the os pubis to the bladder and radiate into the inner longitudinal muscle tracts anteriorly. An outer supplementary longitudinal fiber layer courses in thin layers to the preurethral ligament or to the superior fascia of the urogenital diaphragm. From the posterior aspect of the urethra, radiate longitudinal branches into the vaginal wall. These are intrinsically involved in the formation of the urethrovaginal septum. The circular fiber layer forms the smooth muscle lissosphincter urethrae (Hayek) in the central region of the urethra.

The diagonally striped muscle fibers originate from the deep transverse perineal muscle and form a urethrovaginal sphincter muscle and rhabdosphincter urethrae. In the area of the urethrovaginal septum, the striated muscle bundles of the urethrovaginal sphincter radiate into the vaginal wall.

The adventitia is loosely applied in the upper posterior urethra, whereas it is densely adherent to the fascia vaginalis in the lower urethra within the urethrovaginal septum.

Vessels and Nerves

The arterial vessels originate from the vaginal arteries and from branches of the internal pudendal arteries. Venous drainage is directed toward the pudendal plexus and to the veins of the external genitalia.

The lymphatics reach from the lower urethra to the superficial and deep inguinal lymph nodes. From the upper urethra, they travel along the bladder pillar to the interiliac and the inferior gluteal node groups.

Innervation is from the vesical plexus as well as from the pudendal nerve. The latter carries both motor and sensory fibers.

Anatomical knowledge of the urethra is vital in anterior colporrhaphy (see p. 330), Manchester operation (see p. 462) and repair of vesicovaginal fistula (see p. 666).

RECTUM

The rectum occupies an area from about the level of the second sacral vertebra to the anus. It curves along the sacrum (Figs. 17 and 29) to form the sacral flexure (flexura sacralis) in the pars pelvina; then, in its pars perinealis (canalis perinealis), it arcs anteriorly to yield the perineal flexure (flexura perinealis). In the region of the sacral flexure, the rectum is displaced to the right, while it occupies the midline in the pars perinealis. Immediately above the perineal portion is the ampulla recti.

Layers of the Wall

The architecture of the rectal wall corresponds more or less to that of the large intestine in the pars pelvina. Only the longitudinal

Figure 29.

Blood supply of the rectum. The branches
of the middle sacral artery have been omitted.
1 Rectal ampulla, *2* external anal sphincter
muscle, *3* inferior hemorrhoidal artery, *4*
pelvic diaphragm, *5* internal pudendal artery,
6 middle hemorrhoidal artery, *7* rectosigmoid
artery, *8* Sudeck's point where the rectosigmoid artery takes off from the inferior
mesenteric artery, *9* superior hemorrhoidal
artery (endarterial branch of the inferior
mesenteric artery).

55

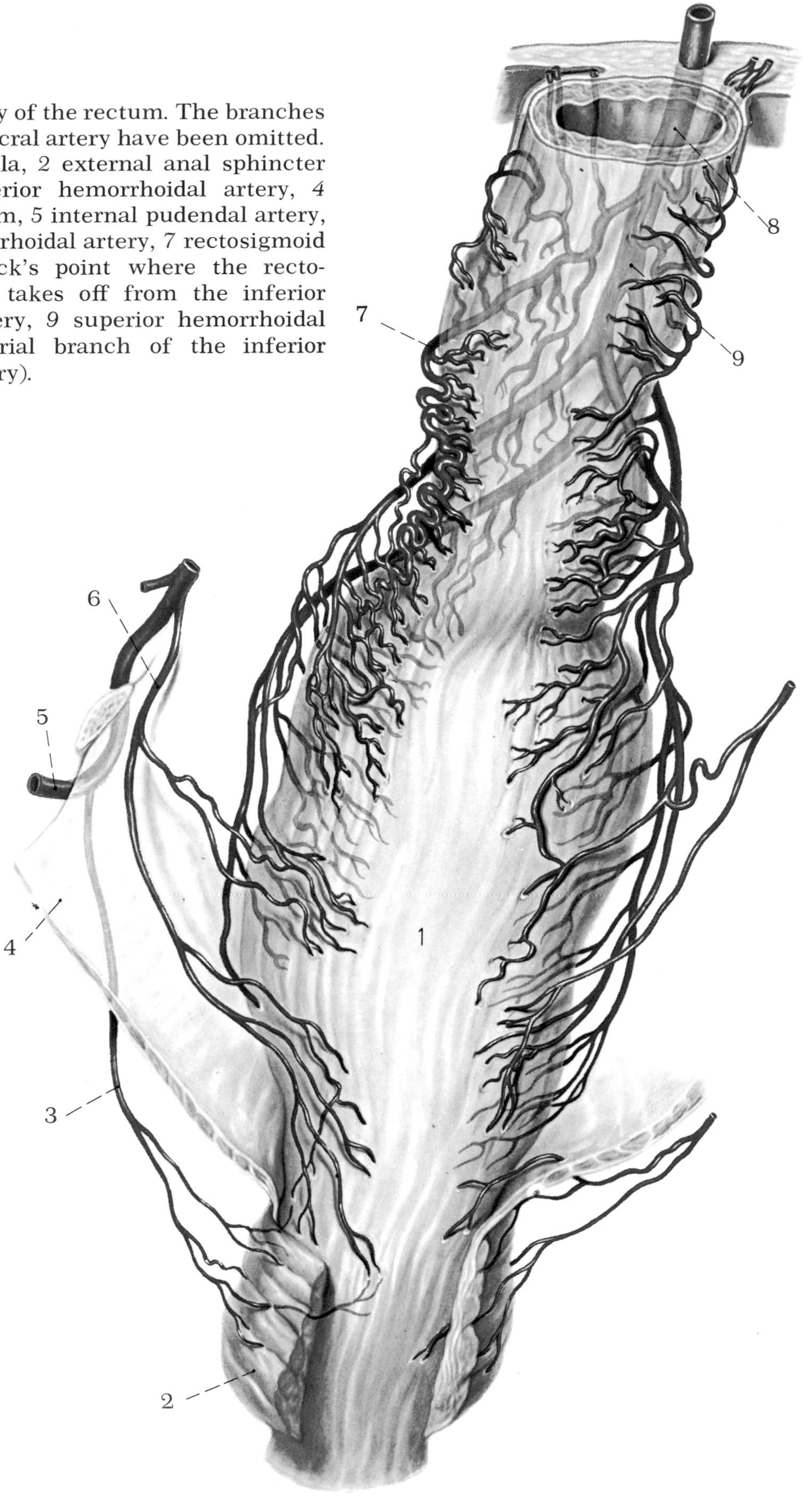

musculature completely and uniformly envelops the rectum in the form of an outer muscle layer. There are but a few (at most three) diagonal folds, the plicae transversalis recti, that can be found in the mucosa. The large fold (the middle one) is named after Kohlrausch. The anal canal (see p. 13) will be discussed in the section on Anus and Anorectal Canal.

Relationships to Adjacent Organs

There is no peritoneum over the posterior wall of the rectum. Loose connective tissue extends from the sides; this lateral connective tissue is called the paraproctium. The anterior rectal wall is connected to posterior wall of the vagina by means of the rectovaginal septum. Three peritoneal pockets are formed above this area. In the middle is the culdesac of Douglas (excavatio rectouterina) and laterally are the fossae pararectales. The anal canal is fixed within the pelvic diaphragm where it is surrounded by the levator ani muscle (see p. 18) and the external anal sphincter muscle (see p. 15).

Vessels and Nerves

With regard to arteries (Fig. 29), the rectum is supplied by the superior hemorrhoidal artery (the arteria rectalis superior arising from the inferior mesenteric artery), the paired middle hemorrhoidal arteries (from the internal iliac arteries) and the paired inferior hemorrhoidal arteries (from the internal pudendal arteries). The middle hemorrhoidal arteries reach the rectum by way of the pararectal connective tissue, specifically the lateral aspect of the rectal pillar; they anastomose with both superior and inferior hemorrhoidal arteries. The superior hemorrhoidal artery, at the dorsal side of the rectum, sends out two main branches, each of which further subdivides into a left and a right branch, respectively. Laterally to the rectum, the uppermost of these branches form anastomoses by means of vascular arcades that originate in the rectosigmoid artery. Where the rectosigmoid artery takes off from the mesenteric ar-

Figure 30.

Innervation of the rectum. *1* Plexus pelvinus (inferior hypogastric plexus), *2* left hypogastrie nerve arising from the superior hypogastric plexus, *3* rectal nerve rami, *4* sympathetic trunk with a ganglion, *5* pelvic nerves from spinal roots S2 and S3 (pelvic splanchnic nerves), *6* pelvic nerve from S4, *7* communication with uterovaginal and vesical plexuses, *8* pudendal nerve, *9* inferior rectal rami, *10* external anal sphincter, *11* median rectal plexus derived from the plexus pelvinus, *12* levator ani muscle, *13* long branch innervating the levator ani muscle.

See illustration on opposite page.

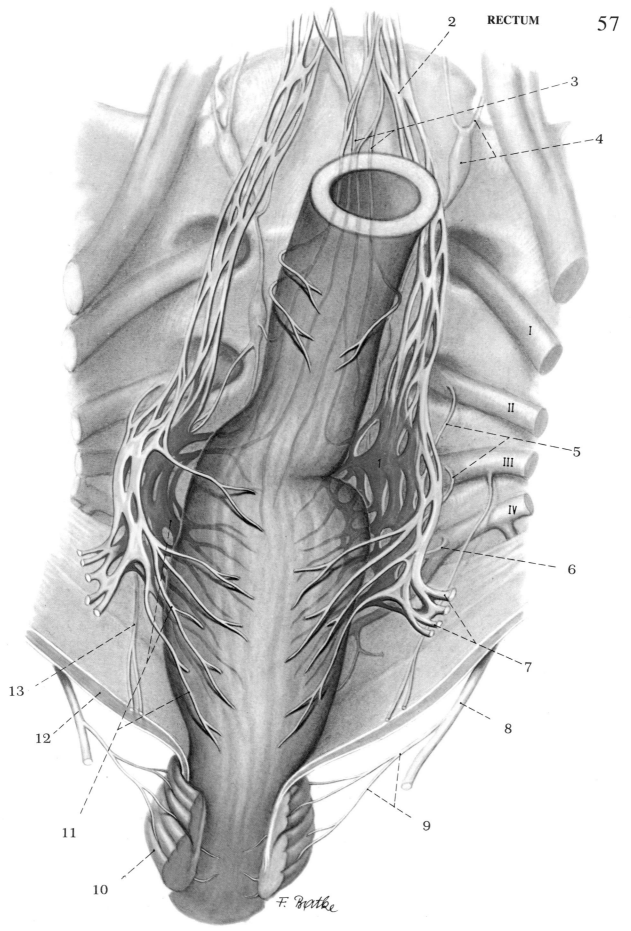

Figure 30. *See legend on opposite page.*

tery is called the "critical point" (Sudeck's point) because it is the last artery that is connected with the other colonic arteries by adequate anastomoses. The middle hemorrhoidal arteries anastomose with the superior hemorrhoidal arteries at the arcades where the two main branches divide. The anastomoses with the inferior hemorrhoidal arteries occur within the muscular layer. Small branches of the middle sacral artery reach the posterior wall of the rectum to just above the pelvic diaphragm.

Blood flowing from the rectum is collected in the superior hemorrhoidal veins (vena rectalis superior), that are formed from the rectal venous plexus (pars superior) situated in the paraproctium. These veins reach the inferior mesenteric vein. From the rectal ampulla, veins also lead to the rectal venous plexus, which, in this location, has connections with the uterine or vaginal venous plexuses, and then, by way of the middle hemorrhoidal veins, to the internal iliac veins. Other veins arise from the dorsal side of the rectum to reach the middle sacral vein and from the inferior hemorrhoidal veins (see p. 15) to the internal pudendal veins. All of these veins are interconnected with each other via the plexus venosus rectalis.

Lymph vessels follow the veins in their course and drain into the rectal, internal iliac, sacral and inguinal lymph node groups (see also p. 15).

The rectum is innervated by the rectal plexus (Fig. 30). The superior rectal plexus represents a continuation of the plexus that accompanies the inferior mesenteric artery. It supplies the portion that connects to sigmoid with both sympathetic and parasympathetic nerves. The superior hypogastric plexus is formed from the lumbar splanchnic nerves of the sympathetic trunk and continues laterally into the hypogastric nerve. The latter develops on either side of the sympathetic root of the pelvic plexus (plexus pelvinus, plexus hypogastricus inferior). The parasympathetic roots of this plexus originate from the sacral region (S2–S4) and reach the plexus by way of the pelvic nerves (nervi pelvici, nervi splanchnici pelvini). The lower portion of the rectum receives both sympathetic and parasympathetic innervation from the median rectal plexus that begins in the pelvic plexus. The pelvic plexus lies within the paraproctium and is connected to the uterovaginal and the vesical plexuses. Sympathetic fibers entwining the rectal arteries also reach the rectum as the inferior rectal plexus. Finally, the external anal sphincter is innervated by means of the inferior rectal nerves that arise from the pudendal nerve.

Intimate knowledge of the anatomical details of the rectum is needed in the performance of radical vaginal surgery (see p. 80), vaginal hysterectomy (see p. 214), colpoperineorrhaphy (see p. 366), procedure for vaginal atresia (see p. 392) and repair of perineal laceration (see p. 531).

PELVIC CONNECTIVE TISSUE

The pelvic connective tissue invests those subperitoneal or extraperitoneal tissues that connect the viscera and the abdominal

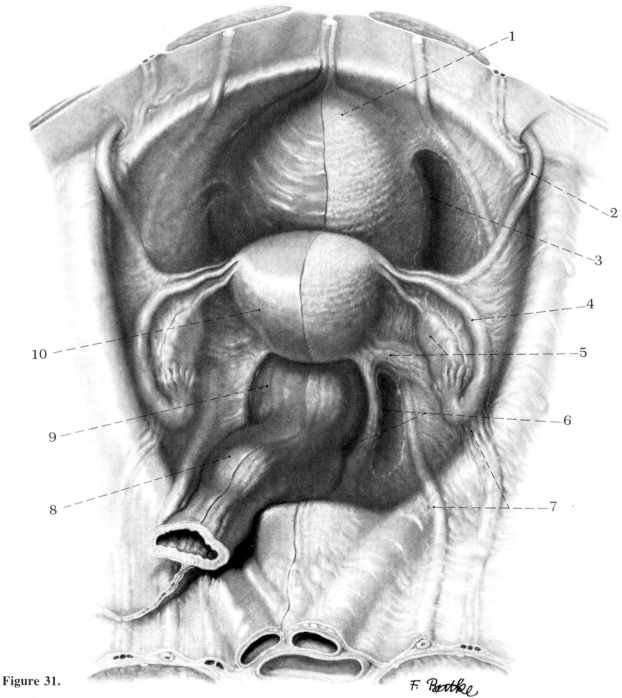

Figure 31.

Connective tissue spaces of the true pelvis as seen from above. The peritoneum has been removed from the left half. *1* Urinary bladder, *2* round ligament, *3* paravesical space, *4* uterine tube, *5* ovary and cardinal ligament, *6* uterosacral ligament and the artificial space created within the paraproctium (the medial portion of the rectal pillar) medially to the ureter, *7* infundibulopelvic ligament and ureter, *8* rectum, *9* excavatio rectouterina, *10* uterus.

wall. In addition to loose areolar tissue, there are denser, fibrous, syndesmotic elements that are reenforced by smooth muscle.

Pelvic connective tissue surrounds the viscera in denser layers

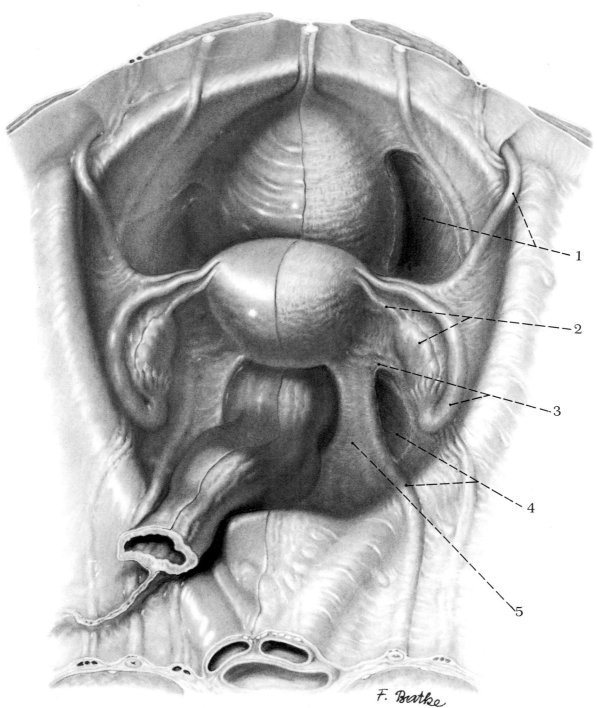

Figure 32.

Connective tissue space of the true pelvis as in Figure 31. *1* Paravesical space and round ligament, *2* utero-ovarian ligament and ovary, *3* cardinal ligament and uterine tube, *4* ureter and artificial space in the lateral aspect of the rectal pillar, *5* medial portion of the rectal pillar.

called adventitia as well as fascia. Laterally to the organs, the connective tissue is arranged to serve as guiding lamellae for vessels and nerves in the paracolpium, parametrium, paracystium and paraproctium leading to specific organs. The anchoring tissues are called bands, muscles and pillars. We are familiar, for instance, with bladder pillars, uterovaginal pillars, cervical pillars and rectal pillars (see Fig. 18). These pillars, of course, do not have any supporting function for the viscera, but they do check organ displacement. Support against pressure from above results only from pelvic floor musculature (see p. 18).

There are large numbers of other terms for pelvic connective tissue and its component parts, such as intrapelvic body, vessel-nerve-guiding lamella, connective-tissue matrix (horizontal and frontal), endopelvic fascia and similar designations. It should be noted, however, that different writers have expounded the same concepts for different structures, adding confusion to an already complicated connective tissue construction. We shall limit ourselves here to the most utilitarian and obvious expressions.

The loose areolar tissue interposed between denser connective tissue strands fills those cavities that can be easily demonstrated during surgery. One differentiates the prevesical, paravesical, pararectal, retrorectal, vesicocervical, vesicovaginal, urethrovaginal and rectovaginal spaces (see Figs. 31 and 32).

Anteriorly, the pelvic connective tissue attaches to the pelvic wall along the arcus tendineus of the pelvic fascia. This border begins near the lower edge of the symphysis pubis and crosses the tendinous arc of the obturator fascia (levator ani muscle) close to the ischial spine to reach the pelvic fascia. The arcus tendineus of the pelvic fascia corresponds to a striped thickening of the superior levator fascia. Anteriorly, between the symphysis and the bladder, is the pubovesical ligament (also called pubovesical muscle) permeated by smooth muscle fibers. This band represents the most anterior part of the anterior border lamella of the pelvic connective tissue. The posterior border lamella is weaker; it belongs to the rectal pillar and reaches the pelvic wall about in the angle of bifurcation of the common iliac artery.

The center of the intrapelvic body is that point at which the connective tissue is most powerfully developed. It is found where the visceral vessels separate from the pelvic wall. Denser strands are developed from this part within the connective tissue as guiding pathways for vessels and nerves. The strongest structure is the uterovaginal pillar. It participates in the formation of the parametrium. Its base is the cardinal ligament (Fig. 33) that connects the cervix with the lateral pelvic wall and is attached to the pelvic floor only with loose areolar tissue. It does continue, however, into the lateral connective tissue of the vagina, that is, into the paracolpium.

As to the cardinal ligament, we should discuss its various designations and interpretations. The term cardinal ligament was first introduced into the literature not by Mackenrodt, but by Kocks in 1880, who spoke of the pars cardinalis ligamentum lati when referring to the basal part of the broad ligament. Mackenrodt, in 1895, characterized the taut connective tissue fibers that stretch from the cervix by the term ligamentum transversale colli or ligamentum

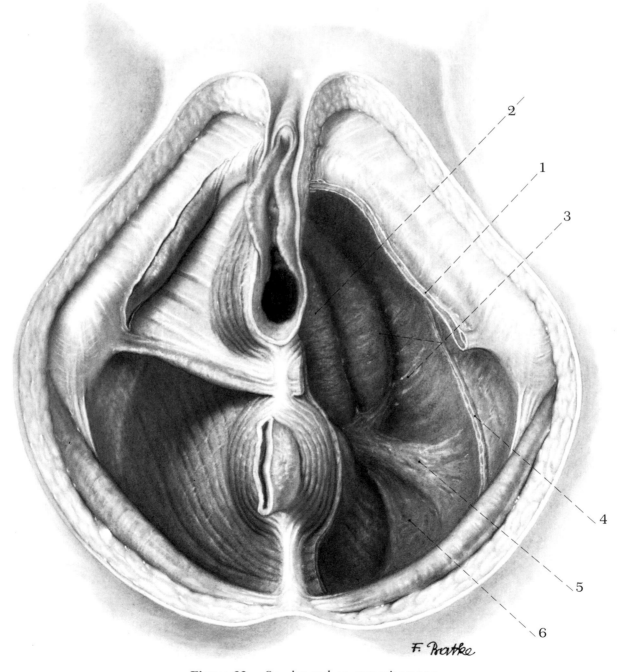

Figure 33.   *See legend on opposite page.*

latum colli. Over the intervening years, since then, other expressions have been used, including pars media retinaculum uteri (Martin, 1911), pars media fasciae pelvis (the same Martin, 1950), tunica vasorum uteri (Pernkopf and Pichler, 1945), and frontal connective tissue (Peham and Amreich, 1930). The terms cervical pillar, cardinal ligament, transverse cervical ligament, and Mackenrodt's ligament can all be considered interchangeably synonymous.

Based on the rules of priority, it would be appropriate to use these several expressions for the connecting structure between the cervix and the pelvic wall, designating the connective tissue lying above it and attached to the corpus uteri as the parametrium.

Augmented connective tissue fibers embedded with smooth muscle fibers are found on the anterior surface of the cardinal ligament. They course laterally near the pelvic wall and medially near the uterus, extending to the vesical fascia. Collectively, these fibers represent the bladder pillar. The medial fibers are also called the vesicouterine ligament. Most of the blood vessels and nerves pass through the lateral portion that reaches the pubovesical ligament (musculus pubovesicalis).

Within the vesicouterine ligament, courses the vesicovaginal artery, a constant finding. This vessel arises from the uterine artery (variously). Between the medial and lateral parts of the bladder pillar, is encountered loose areolar tissue. All the connective tissue lying laterally to the bladder, including the loose areolar tissue, is called the paracystium.

Dorsally, the rectal pillar stretches from the cardinal ligament to the rectum. The rectal pillars bow rather far laterally because the space of Douglas descends between their medial aspects. At these medial borders are the uterosacral ligaments (ligamentum rectouterinum or sacrouterinum). They represent the connective tissue base of the plicae rectouterinae, the peritoneal folds of which form the lateral border of the culdesac of Douglas. The lateral aspect of the rectal pillar originates from the dorsal part of the cardinal ligament and contains vessels and nerves. The ureter is found between these checkrein ligaments embedded in its connective tissue sheath (ureteral lamina). Loose areolar tissue fills the surrounding spaces. Obviously, the entire investing tissue around the rectum can be designated the paraproctium.

The urinary, genital and digestive tracts are all interconnected

---

Figure 33.

Pelvic connective tissue viewed from below with the left half of the urogenital and pelvic diaphragms removed. *1* Cut edge of urogenital diaphragm, *2* vagina with vaginal fascia, *3* urinary bladder with the vesical fascia, paracystium, *4* cut edge of pelvic diaphragm, *5* cardinal ligament, *6* paraproctium.

See illustration on opposite page.

in the midline by connective tissue infiltrated with smooth muscle. Included in this structure are the urethrovaginal septum (see p. 27), the rectovaginal septum (see p. 27) and the supravaginal septum (see p. 52).

FASCIAL SPACES

The connective tissue spaces are filled with loose areolar tissue that can easily be entered by blunt dissection during surgery. In this way the various spaces can be demonstrated.

Paravesical and Prevesical Spaces (Figs. 31, 32 and 34)

The paravesical space is found laterally to the bladder and the anterior aspect of the formed connective tissue that constitutes the bladder pillar. It is bordered behind by the root of the bladder pillar from the center of the intrapelvic body, and by the base of the cardinal ligament, extending to the lateral pelvic wall. Anteriorly, the paravesical space communicates with the prevesical space, which connects, in turn, with the paravesical space of the opposite side. The prevesical space is occluded below by the pubovesical ligaments. The paravesical and prevesical spaces represent parts of the overlying preperitoneal space of Retzius.

Pararectal Space (Figs. 31, 32 and 34)

This space is bordered laterally by the pelvic wall and anterolaterally by the posterior edge of the cardinal ligament or its root, which consists of the center of the intrapelvic body. The medial border is the rectal pillar. Caudally, it reaches to the pelvic floor.

The ureter progresses in its connective tissue sheath, the ureteral lamella, through the rectal pillar. The medial part of the rectal pillar is formed from the uterosacral ligament; vessels and nerves course through its lateral aspect. It contains loose connective tissue. In a surgical preparation it is possible to enter from above between the rectal pillar borders so as to create spaces that are medial and lateral to the ureter and the ureteral fold (Figs. 31 and 32), but that do not actually represent the pararectal space. The spaces lie within the rectal pillars. If one enters between the borders of the rectal pillars, one can advance up to the rectovaginal space.

Medially, the pararectal space is separated from the retrorectal space by the uterosacral ligament. The pararectal space communicates with the paravesical space beneath the cardinal ligament because, as mentioned earlier, the cardinal ligament is attached dor-

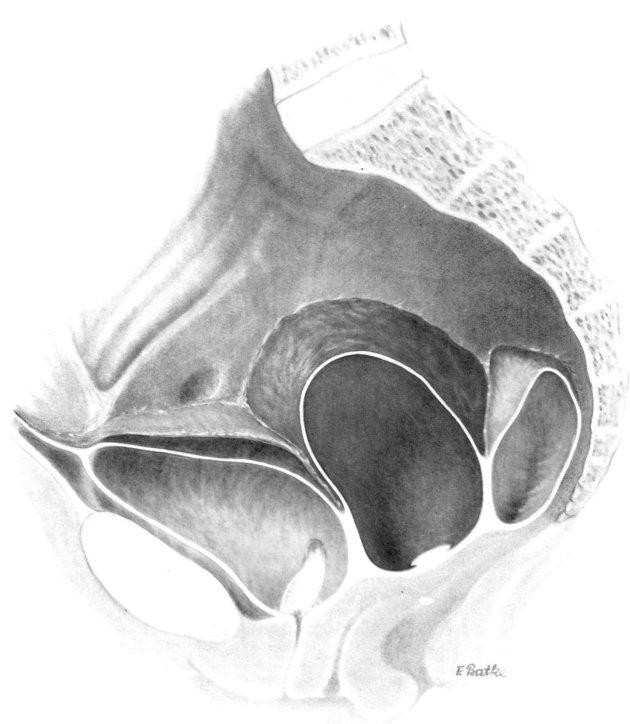

Figure 34.

Median sagittal section of the lateral connective tissue spaces, shown schematically as artificially created. *Blue,* paravesical space; *red,* connective tissue space lateral to the uterus; *green,* pararectal space.

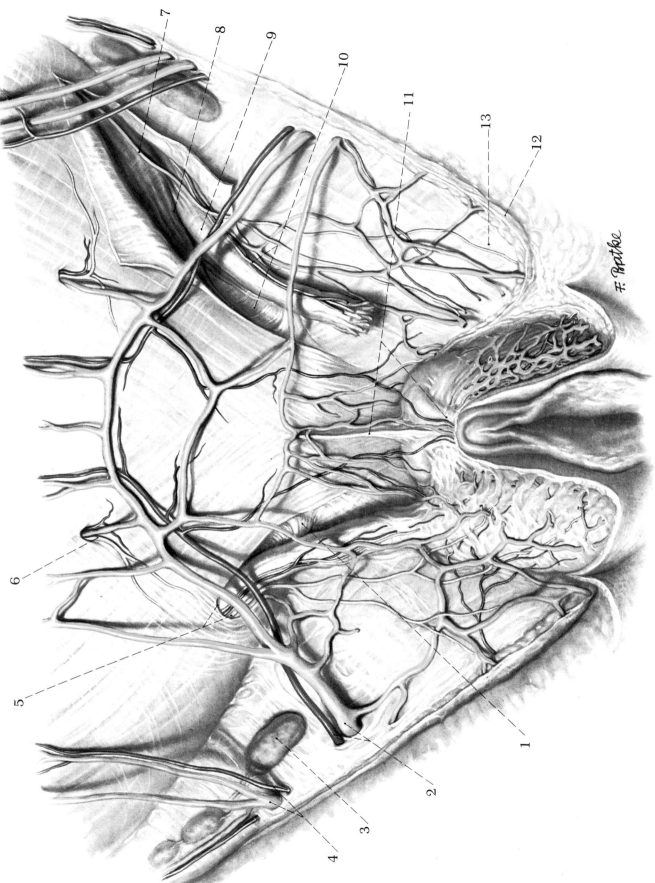

Figure 35.   *See legend on opposite page.*

The lateral crus ends together with the inguinal ligament at the pubic tuberculum, while the medial crus forms the posterior wall of the external inguinal ring as the reflex inguinal ligament (Colles) and attaches at the superior ramus of the pubis.

The round ligament (ligamentum teres uteri, ligamentum rotundum) exits through the inguinal canal accompanied by blood and lymph vessels (see p. 34) and radiates into the connective tissue of the labium majus (see Fig. 35). It is associated with the ilioinguinal nerve and the genital ramus of the genitofemoral nerve. The latter nerves supply the skin in the area of the labium majus (see p. 7) and the adjoining inner surface of the thigh. Preperitoneal adipose tissue (Imlach's fat pad) becomes visible in the external inguinal ring next to the round ligament. The external inguinal ring represents a site of minimal resistance for the anterior abdominal wall.

The inguinal canal (see Fig. 35) is bounded caudally by the inguinal ligament, cranially by the lower edges of the transverse abdominal muscle and of the internal oblique abdominal muscle. The anterior surface is formed of the aponeurosis of the external oblique abdominal muscle; the posterior wall is the transversalis fascia, strengthened by the interfoveolar ligament.

For additional anatomical details the reader is referred to appropriate anatomy sources. Knowledge of the anatomy of this area is especially important in the operative treatment of vulvar carcinoma (see p. 624).

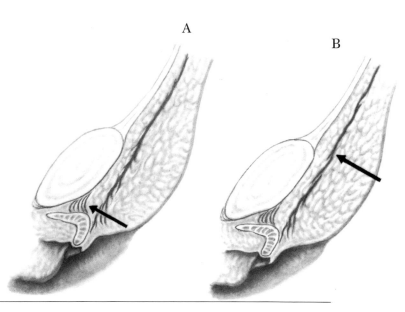

Figure 36.

A, Median sagittal section through the anterior abdominal wall to illustrate the suspensory ligament of the clitoris (arrow). *B,* Similar diagrammatic representation showing Camper's fascia (arrow) which terminates caudally in the ligamentum fundiforme clitoridis.

Figure 35.

Pubic and inguinal regions. The inguinal ring on the right is sharply delimited; the left inguinal canal has been opened and the round ligament divided. *1* Ligamentum inguinale reflexum, *2* external pudendal artery and vein, *3* superficial inguinal lymph node, *4* superficial epigastric artery and vein, *5* external inguinal ring and ilioinguinal nerve, *6* iliohypogastric nerve, *7* ilioinguinal nerve, *8* caudal edge of internal oblique abdominal muscle, *9* round ligament, *10* transversalis fascia and genital nerve ramus, *11* suspensory ligament of the clitoris and corpus clitoridis, *12* connective tissue lamella (Camper's fascia), *13* fascia lata.

See illustration on opposite page.

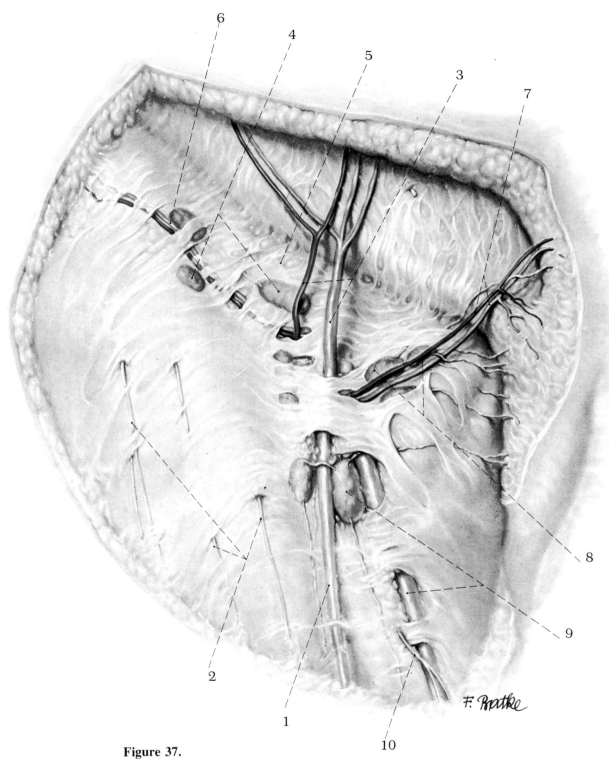

Figure 37.

Subinguinal region demonstrating the subcutaneous layer with its coarse connective tissue (previously designated superficial femoral fascia). *1* accessory saphenous vein (lateral to the greater saphenous vein), *2* branches of the lateral femoral cutaneous nerve, *3* superficial epigastric artery and vein, *4* superficial inguinal lymph nodes (horizontal tract), *5* subcutaneous connective tissue, *6* superficial circumflex iliac artery and vein, *7* external pudendal vessels, *8* superficial inguinal lymph nodes (horizontal tract), *9* greater saphenous vein and superficial inguinal nodes (vertical tract), *10* anterior cutaneous femoral nerve ramus.

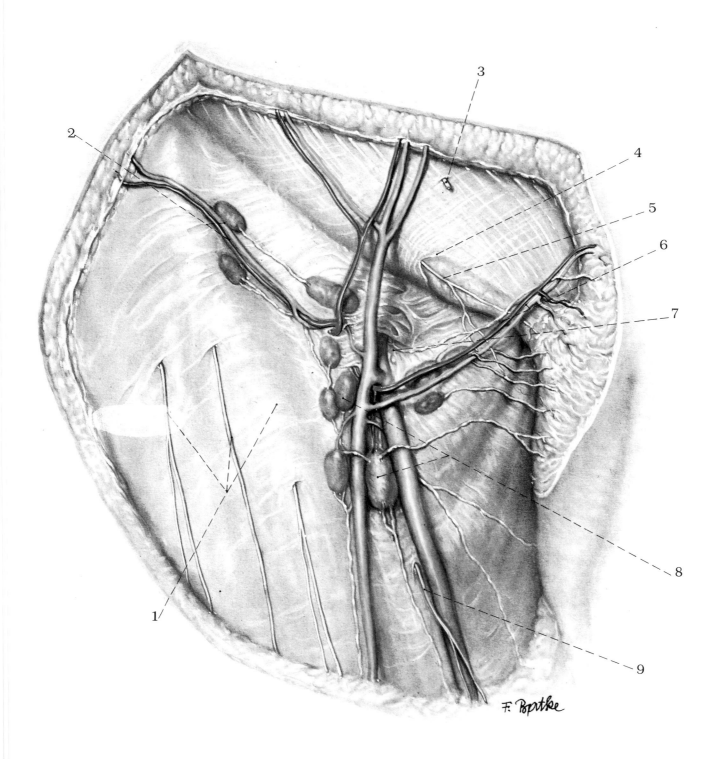

Figure 38.

Inguinal and subinguinal regions and fascia lata. *1* Fascia lata and branches of lateral femoral cutaneous nerve, *2* superficial circumflex iliac vessels, *3* iliohypogastric nerve, *4* external inguinal ring, *5* ilioinguinal nerve, *6* external pudendal artery and vein, *7* fascia cribrosa, *8* superficial inguinal lymph nodes (vertical tract), *9* anterior femoral cutaneous ramus.

strengthened by the falx inguinalis. The lateral border is formed by the arcus iliopectineus (ligamentum interlacunare, ligamentum iliopectineum) stretching between the inguinal ligament and the iliopubic eminence (eminentia iliopectinea).

The femoral artery, vein and lymphatics pass through the lacuna vasorum in a medial direction. The medial portion of the vascular orifice corresponds to the femoral canal, the inner opening of which (the anulus femoralis) is closed off by a loose septum, the femoral septum (Cloquet).

Lacuna Musculorum

The muscular orifice that is joined laterally to the lacuna vasorum is bordered in front by the inguinal ligament, medially by the arcus iliopectineus, and posterolaterally by the iliac portion of the innominate bone (os coxae). Through it pass the iliopsoas muscle with its fascial covering and the medially coassociated femoral nerve. Laterally, immediately adjacent to the anterior superior iliac spine, courses the lateral femoral cutaneous nerve.

Operative treatment of vulvar carcinoma (see p. 624) demands intimate anatomical knowledge of this region.

OPERATIVE
TECHNIQUE

SCHAUTA-AMREICH RADICAL VAGINAL HYSTERECTOMY FOR CARCINOMA OF THE CERVIX

SCHUCHARDT INCISION

A sufficiently large vaginal opening for access to the pelvic structures is achieved by means of a left-sided Schuchardt incision of the perineum and levator. Bilateral incisions are almost never necessary for exposure to the operative field. The perineal-levator incision opens the left pararectal space while simultaneously divid-

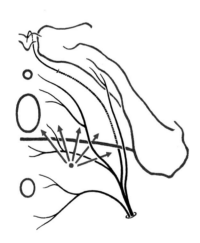

Figure 43.

Schauta-Amreich procedure. Infiltration of the Schuchardt incision site begins with perineal infiltration of a fan-shaped area with physiologic saline solution. The surgeon's left index finger is inserted into the vagina to palpate the ischial tuberosity. A long needle is inserted about 3 cm. to the left of the anus and advanced close to the ischial tuberosity while he simultaneously injects the fluid. Diagram above shows how the branches of the pudendal nerve are infiltrated during the fan-shaped infiltration (red) of the solution.

See illustration on opposite page.

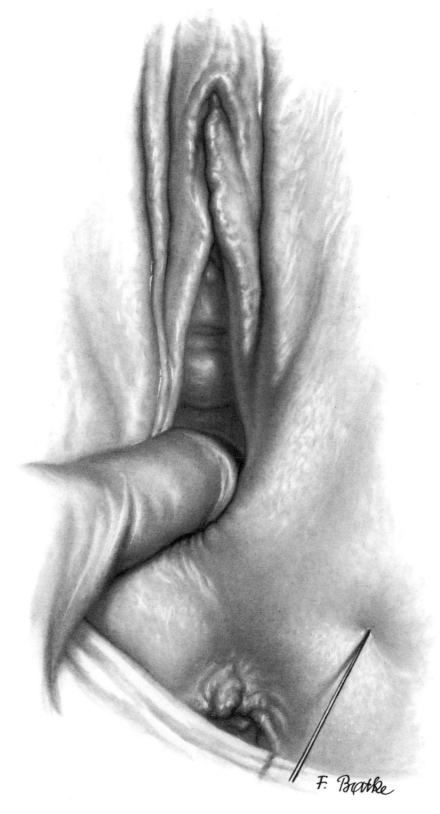

Figure 43. *See legend on opposite page.*

F. Bratke

ing the horizontal pelvic fascia on the left. This latter dense connective tissue septum separates the pararectal and paravesical spaces; dividing this septum unites both spaces alongside the bladder and the rectum. To complete the preparation of these spaces one can gently and bluntly dissect the yielding connective tissue fibers in the paravesical and pararectal spaces with a finger until one has reached up the pelvic wall next to the bladder and the rectum.

Correct dissection of the "para spaces" is critically important for successful execution of the radical vaginal operation. One can reach these spaces with impunity if one first infiltrates the tissues with fluid.

Infiltration of the Incision Sites

The perineum and vagina are infiltrated locally with physiologic saline solution for hemostatic purposes. One may consider the possibility of adding vasoconstrictor agents such as a dilute solution containing 5 drops of vasopressin per 100 cc. Subfascial injection of the left vaginal wall and the site of the mucosal circumcision will lift the vaginal wall from the rectum and the bladder, making the longitudinal and circumferential electrocautery incisions relatively safe with little likelihood of injury to adjacent structures.

Figure 44.

Schauta-Amreich procedure. Infiltration of the Schuchardt incision site continues with the needle being advanced subcutaneously up to the posterior commissure. This is done after the perineum has been thoroughly infiltrated.

See illustration on opposite page.

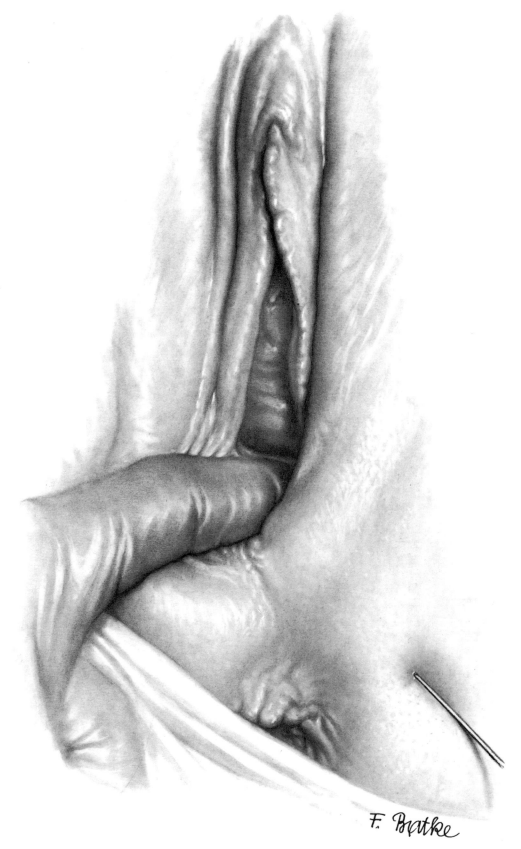

Figure 44.   *See legend on opposite page.*

amounts are administered at 12, 3, 6 and 9 o'clock, respectively (Fig. 47). For selecting the appropriate distance of the puncture sites from the portio, one must take into account the size of the primary tumor of the cervix. Infiltration of the vaginal wall should be 3–4 cm. distal from the edge of the carcinoma because it is essential to perform the vaginal circumcision in an area of healthy vaginal tissue that is grossly free of tumor.

Details of the Schuchardt Incision

SITE.   The perineal incision begins at the posterior commissure three fingerbreadths to the left of the midline and curves around the anus toward the ischial tuberosity (Fig. 48). The lower end of the incision is carried to the level of the anus. The incision is then extended up from the posterior commissure into the left vaginal wall cephalad to the future site of the circular vaginal circumcision.

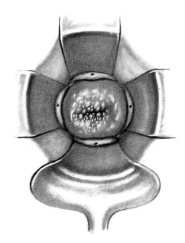

Figure 46.

 Schauta-Amreich procedure. Infiltration of the site of the vaginal circumcision. The vagina is completely exposed with four retractors, including one posterior leaf-shaped and three right-angled spatulas. The needle is inserted at 12 o'clock in the anterior vaginal fornix about 3 cm. from the portio; 20 cc. of fluid is injected. Inset illustrates the infiltration sites (red) after injection of 20 cc. amounts at 12, 6, 9 and 3 o'clock in the anterior, posterior and lateral fornices.

See illustration on opposite page.

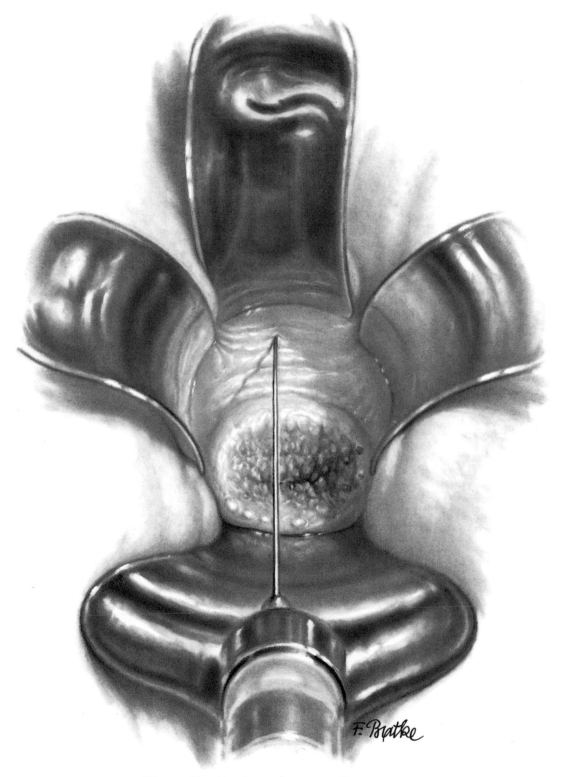

Figure 46. *See legend on opposite page.*

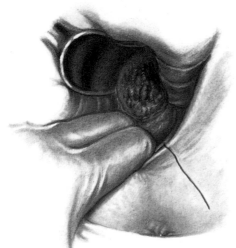

Figure 47.

Schauta-Amreich procedure. Placement of the Schuchardt incision in the perineal skin site. The vagina is stretched by an anterior spatula (held by the right assistant), by the right index finger of the left assistant and by the second and third fingers of the surgeon's left hand. The incision begins at the posterior commissure 3 fingerbreadths to the left of the midline and curves to the left to reach the level of the anus.

Figure 48.

Schauta-Amreich procedure. Extension of the Schuchardt incision up the lateral vaginal wall. The left assistant pushes the left lateral vaginal wall firmly upward with his index finger. The surgeon's left index finger strongly pulls the posterior vaginal wall downward. The right assistant elevates the right vaginal wall to the right with a spatula. The perineal skin is divided and the left vaginal wall is incised up to the lateral fornix.

See illustration on opposite page.

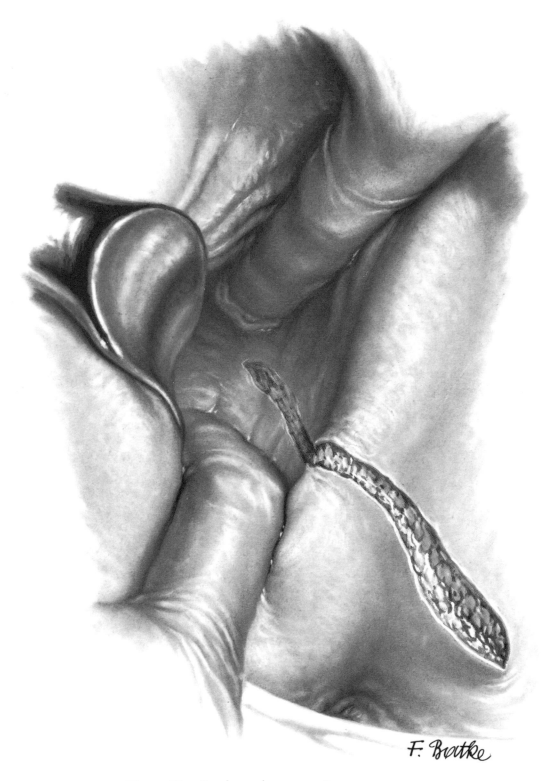

Figure 48. *See legend on opposite page.*

2. Opening the pararectal and the paravesical spaces is rendered more difficult if only lateral fibers of the levator muscles are divided during the electrocautery scoring of the levator ani muscles, leaving the medial puborectal fibers intact. Moreover, when the dissection of the paravesical space is extended too far caudally, the intact upper puborectal fibers of the levator adhere to the bladder pillar, making this structure unduly thick. Later, when it becomes necessary to lay open the ureter, this step is made more complicated as a consequence.

3. If the left vaginal wall incision is made too far medially, one can injure the rectum or the larger pararectal veins. If too lateral, the incision may lacerate the larger veins of the bulbocavernous plexus, although hemostasis is easy to accomplish here.

For details of the relevant anatomy, one should review sections dealing with the external genitalia (see p. 2), the perineum (see p. 8) and the pelvic floor (see p. 18).

Figure 51.

Schauta-Amreich procedure. Opening the left paravesical space. The right assistant retracts the right vaginal wall to the right with an anterior spatula. In the exposed left paravesical space is a spatula held by the left-sided assistant. The pararectal and paravesical spaces have been widely opened on the left and joined. The bladder is visible anteriorly in the depths of the vaginal incision and the rectum is seen posteriorly.

See illustration on opposite page.

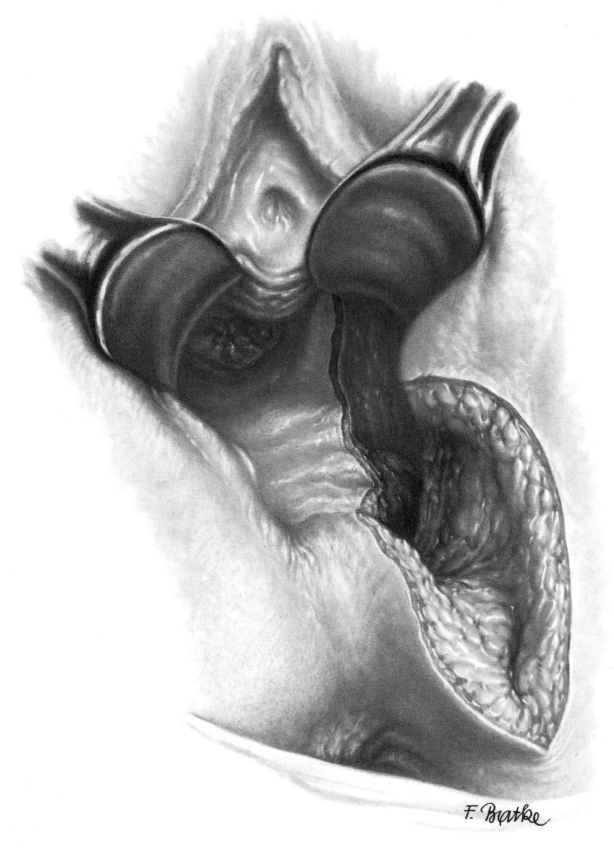

F. Bratke

Figure 51. *See legend on opposite page.*

CIRCUMCISION OF THE VAGINAL CANAL

Site of the Incision

The vaginal circumcision is done in a site selected according to the extent of the carcinoma. It should be placed so that at least 3 cm. of macroscopically healthy vaginal tissue intervenes between the edge of the tumor and the incision.

Technique of the Circumcision

The Schuchardt incision is draped with a gauze sponge that is secured at the lateral wound edges with several silk sutures. The vagina is completely exposed by retractors: the right side is retracted anterolaterally by the right-side assistant, the left vaginal wall is pulled laterally by the left-side assistant, and the posterior wall is depressed by a self-retaining weighted speculum.

The vaginal canal is grasped at the predetermined site anteriorly with several single-toothed tenacula. Then it is grasped more posteriorly with additional tenacula applied in a circular manner (Fig. 52). The vaginal cuff is painted with Lugol's solution to ensure that the circumcision is carried out in mucosa that is entirely healthy.

Figure 52.

Schauta-Amreich procedure. Circumcision of the vaginal canal. The mucosa is stretched by two lateral spatulas and a self-retaining posterior retractor. The left-sided Schuchardt incision wound has been draped with a gauze pad. The portio is first stained with Lugol's solution; 4 cm. of the vagina are designated as the appropriate operative site here. Then the vaginal cuff is grasped with single-toothed tenacula at the preselected 4 cm. distance from the portio. The uppermost wound angle of the longitudinal incision is seen on the left, reaching to the level at which the vaginal circumcision will be carried out.

See illustration on opposite page.

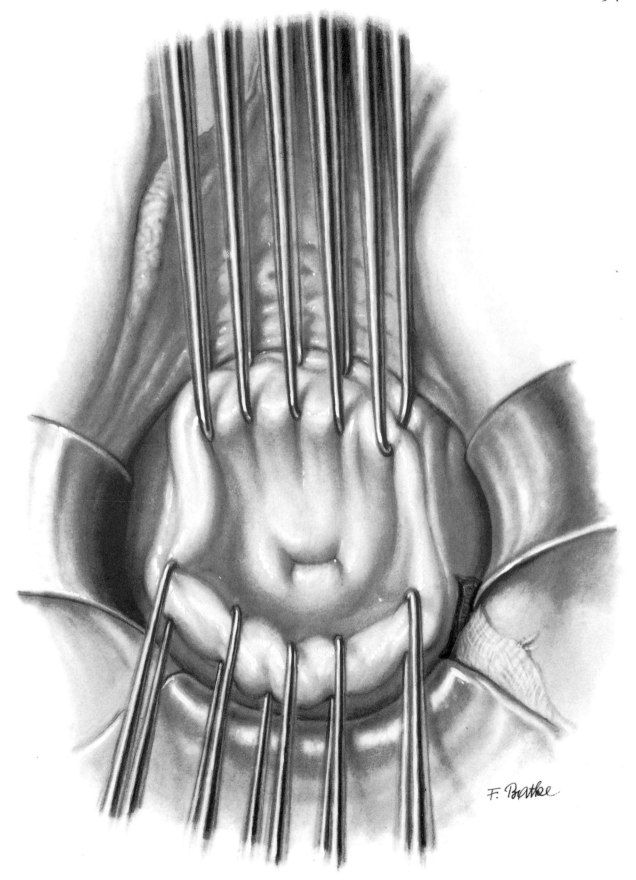

Figure 52. *See legend on opposite page.*

One first circumcises the anterior vaginal wall. To accomplish this, the operator pulls downward on all the tenacula with his left hand, while the right-side assistant retracts and stretches the anterior wall strongly upward with a spatula. The surgeon applies the angulated tip of the electrocautery knife perpendicularly to the stretched vaginal wall and cuts it in a semicircle (Fig. 53). After the anterior circumcision is completed, the assistant on the right grasps the tenacula from the operator and retracts them upward. The left assistant depresses the posterior spatula downward with his left hand, stretching the posterior vaginal wall. The surgeon grasps the posterior vaginal mucosa distally to the tenacula sites with tissue forceps and applies gentle traction to the wall. By doing so, he lifts the vagina somewhat from the rectum. Now the posterior half of the circumcision is carried out above the forceps with the electrocautery knife (Fig. 54).

Figure 53.

Schauta-Amreich procedure. Anterior circumcision of the vagina. The right assistant pushes the anterior vaginal wall vigorously upward with an anterior spatula to stretch the inverted anterior mucosa. Both lateral spatulas retract the vaginal wall apart. The posterior self-retaining retractor has been inserted to depress the posterior wall in a caudal direction. The surgeon pulls the tenacula downward and begins to circumcise the anterior vaginal wall with an angled electrocautery knife closely above the tenacula. The vaginal mucosa and fascia are separated; one can recognize when the correct depth is reached by the wide gaping of the wound caused by spatula pressure.

See illustration on opposite page.

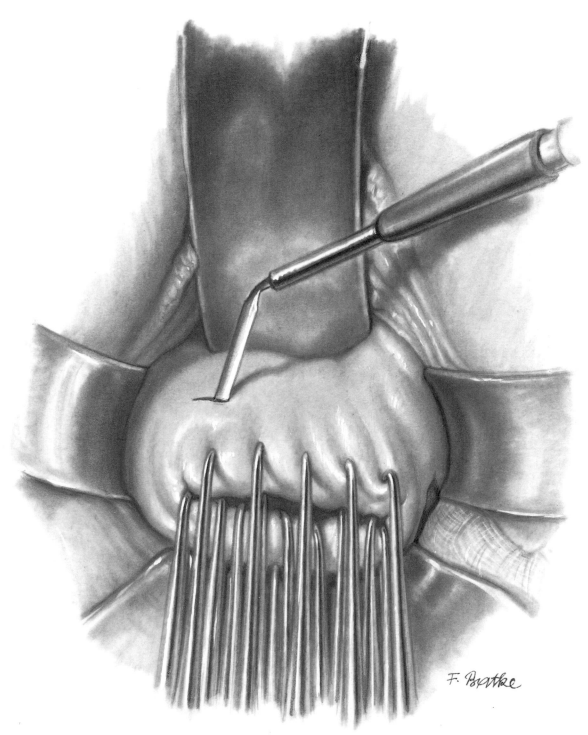

Figure 53. *See legend on opposite page.*

The vaginal circumcision is correctly accomplished when it meets the upper angle of the left vaginal incision wound. In order to avoid rectal injury later, the rectum is further separated from the posterior vaginal wall with curved dissecting scissors (pointed upward) and pushed down (Fig. 55). The rectum, thus mobilized far caudally, is retracted posteriorly with a small gauze strip that is placed under the edge of the self-retaining retractor.

Technical Problems

1. The downward pull of the tenacula that are placed on the anterior vaginal wall does not necessarily stretch the anterior mucosa uniformly so that it may undulate lengthwise. This is especially seen if the vaginal canal is wide and many tenacula have to be used. Under these circumstances, half of the tenacula should be pulled

Figure 54.

Schauta-Amreich procedure. Posterior circumcision. The right assistant pulls the tenacula upward with his left hand. Both assistants retract the lateral vaginal walls to the side with lateral spatulas; a self-retaining retractor depresses the posterior wall. The surgeon grasps the inverted posterior vaginal mucosa with tissue forceps, stretching the vaginal wall with a downward pull. The vagina is circumcised just caudad to the tenacula with electrocautery.

See illustration on opposite page.

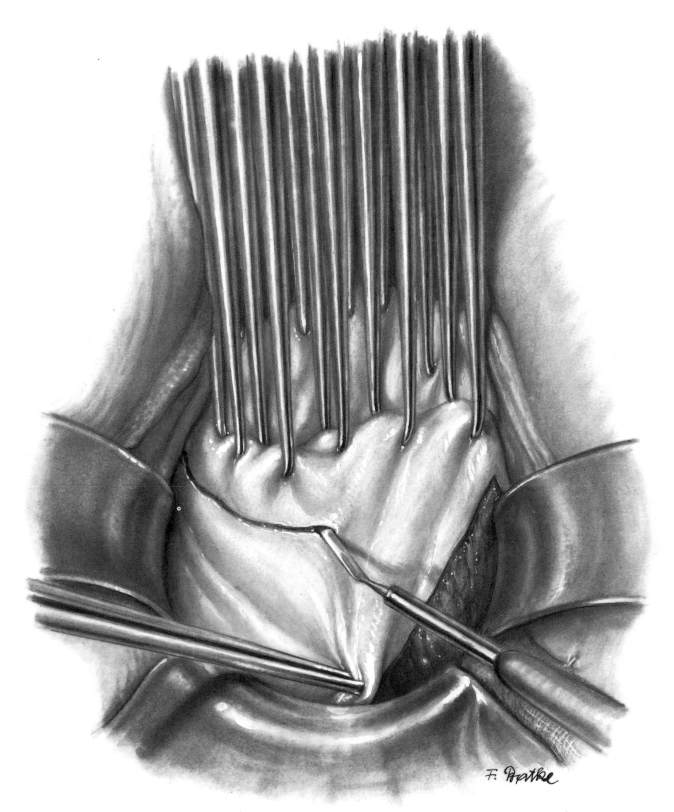

Figure 54. *See legend on opposite page.*

down and to the right by the operator's left hand, and the other half pulled down and to the left with the free left hand of the left-side assistant. The anterior vaginal wall is thus stretched flat without folds.

2. If the circular incision is made too deeply, the vaginal cuff may be perforated at the anterior fornix.

3. If the assistant on the right does not lift the anterior vaginal wall upward with sufficient strength during the anterior circumcision, the vaginal wall will not gape adequately and the bladder may as a consequence be endangered by any further surgical separation.

4. Dissection of the bladder pillar subsequently may be made more difficult if the vaginal canal has not been divided precisely at its lateral margin.

For details of the anatomy of relevant structures, one should review the chapter on the vagina (see p. 24).

Figure 55.

Schauta-Amreich procedure. Forming the vaginal cuff and dissecting the rectum. The vagina is placed on stretch with retractors and the tenacula are raised up by the right-side assistant's left hand. Vaginal circumcision is completed in the same layer and depth posteriorly as it had been done anteriorly. The surgeon pulls the vaginal circumcision wound edge, together with the attached rectum, caudally with the toothed forceps. At the same time, he pushes down on the taut retrocervical connective tissue with the slightly opened dissecting scissors, curved tips pointed upward. This maneuver moves the rectum away.

See illustration on opposite page.

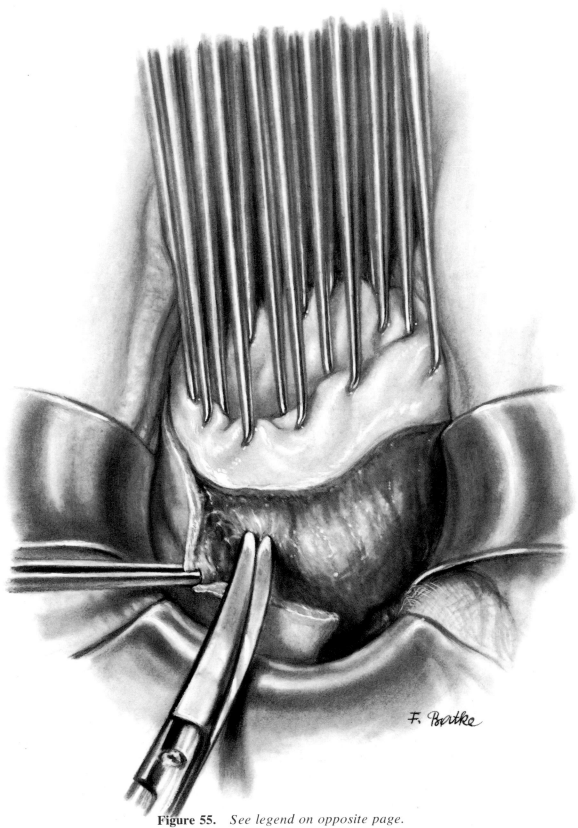

Figure 55. *See legend on opposite page.*

FORMATION OF THE VAGINAL CUFF

Closing the Vaginal Stump

After the vaginal circumcision is completed, the proximal vaginal portion is closed over the cervical carcinoma using mouse-toothed clamps (Fig. 56). Substituting heavy silk sutures instead of these clamps has not been shown to be particularly advantageous because the long ends, when used for continuous traction, can become confused with the long ends of the catgut sutures placed on the ligaments, thus delaying the progress of the operation. Moreover, since the clamps can be held together in the palm of the assistant's hand so that they are parallel to each other, the closed vaginal stump can be directed more exactly and moved like a broad band.

Figure 56.

Schauta-Amreich procedure. Forming the vaginal cuff by substituting mouse-toothed clamps for the tenacula. The vagina is stretched by three retractors. The right assistant elevates the bladder with an anterior spatula and pulls the tenacula down to the right. In a stepwise manner, the surgeon removes the tenacula from the circumcised vagina and grasps the anterior and posterior incision edges of the vaginal stump with mouse-toothed clamps. At the left, the vaginal canal has already been closed with two such clamps. Additional clamps are placed close to the circumferentially severed vaginal canal to form a vaginal cuff.

See illustration on opposite page.

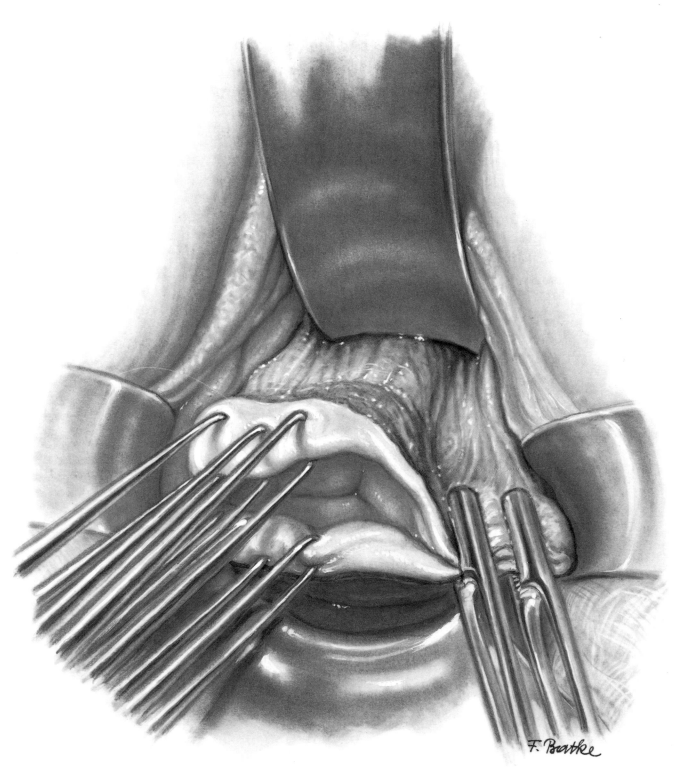

Figure 56. *See legend on opposite page.*

fold. To correct this error one should locate the site of the lower bladder pole with a probe inserted into the bladder through the urethra. This will show that the dissection has been done too near the cervix.

Details of the anatomy relative to this part of the procedure are presented in the sections on vagina (see p. 24), urinary bladder (see p. 47), and pelvic connective tissue spaces (see p. 58).

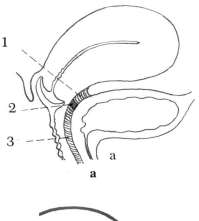

1. loose connective tissue in the vesicocervical space between the uterus and urinary bladder.
2. septum supravaginale
3. loose connective tissue between vaginal and vesical fascias and between vaginal and urethral fascias in the vesicovaginal and urethrovaginal spaces, respectively.

1. vesicouterine space
2. supravaginal septum
3. vesicouterine ligament
4. cardinal ligament
5. rectouterine ligament
6. rectouterine space

Figure 57.

Schauta-Amreich procedure. Dividing the supravaginal septum and opening the vesicocervical space. Three retractors spread the vagina and the right assistant lifts the bladder gently upward with an anterior spatula in his left hand. The left assistant pulls the vaginal cuff down with the mouse-toothed clamps. The surgeon lifts the lower bladder pole with toothed forceps and dissects the stretched fibers of the supravaginal septum near the cervix with scissors. The supravaginal septum and its anatomical relationships are shown diagrammatically in the lateral (a) and coronal (b) cross-sections above.

See illustration on opposite page.

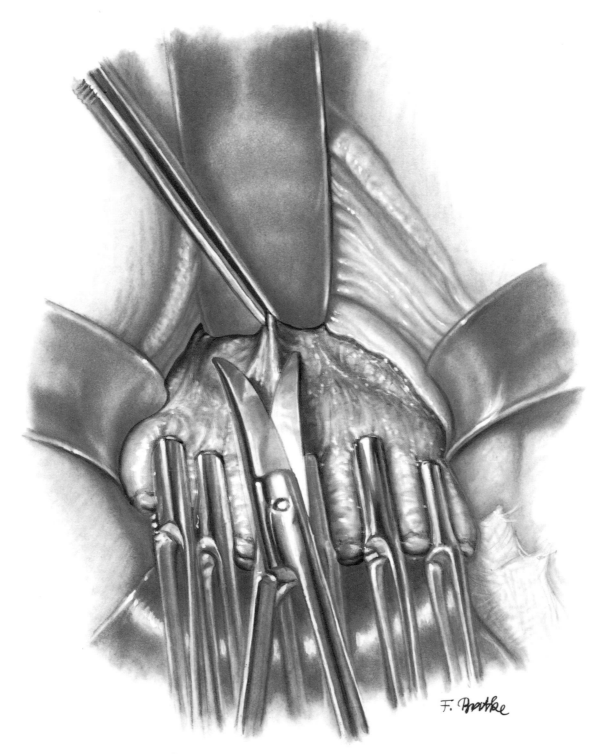

Figure 57. *See legend on opposite page.*

upward. The left assistant places a spatula laterally to the bladder pillar into the left paravesical space and displaces the bladder and the left vaginal wall up and to the left. As a consequence the left bladder pillar is stretched in a sagittal plane (Fig. 58).

The surgeon palpates the stretched bladder pillar with a scissor-like grasp of his second and third fingers. Letting the bladder pillar glide through his fingers, he can identify the ureter in it as a coarse cylindrical cord (Fig. 59), which may pop through his fingertips.

Freeing the Ureter in the Bladder Pillar

The pelvic segment of the ureter first courses down and then bends upward in the bladder pillar before it enters the bladder. The ureteral knee that results from this change in its course can be exactly located in the bladder pillar by palpation. Under normal cir-

Figure 59.

Schauta-Amreich procedure. Locating the ureter in the bladder pillar by palpation. The left bladder pillar is positioned by appropriate spatula pressures. By means of palpation with his second and third fingers, the surgeon locates the ureteral knee in the bladder pillar, allowing the structure to glide through his fingers. If the pillar is not too thick and the palpation is done correctly, the ureteral knee springs audibly across the fingertips.

See illustration on opposite page.

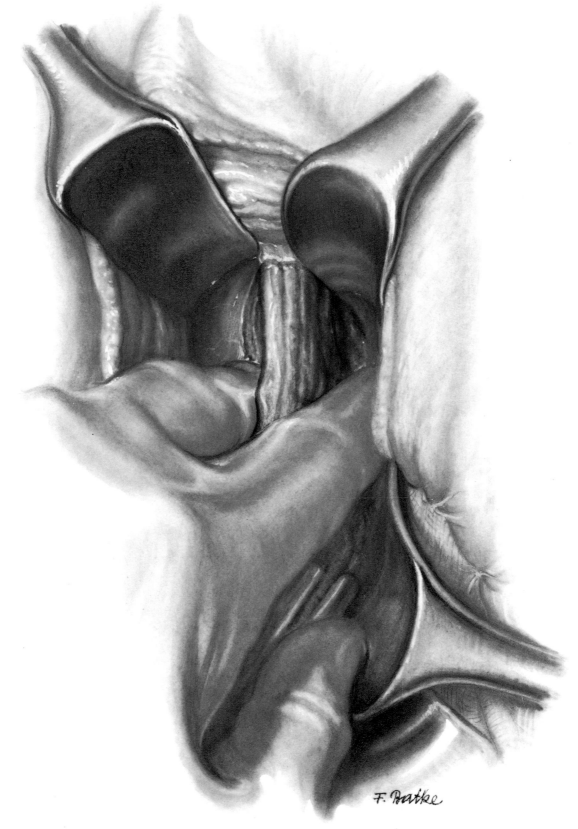

Figure 59. *See legend on opposite page.*

cumstances it is found in the cranial portion of the bladder pillar. Therefore, the caudal part of the pillar can be divided with scissors from the anterior wall of the cervix with no risk of ureteral injury.

Technique for Freeing the Left Ureter

The assistant on the right retracts the vaginal cuff down and to the right. With a spatula inserted anteriorly into the vesicocervical space, he pulls the bladder strongly up and to the right. The left-side assistant places a narrow spatula into the paravesical space

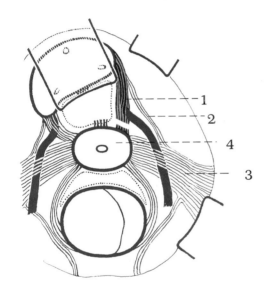

1 — vesicouterine ligament
2 — lateral portion of the bladder pillar
3 — cardinal ligament
4 — cervix

Figure 60.

Schauta-Amreich procedure. Dissection of the bladder pillar from the cervix. The anterior spatulas stretch the bladder pillar by applying upward pressure while they are somewhat tilted. The left assistant still holds back the rectum with the posterolateral spatula. The surgeon pushes the anterior cervical wall caudally with his left middle finger; this stretches the bladder pillar even more, exposing its juncture at the edge of the cervix. One can recognize the tongue-like peritoneal reflection reaching down on the anterior surface of the uterus. The fibers of the bladder pillar are cut close to the cervix. The tips of the scissors should point to the cervix here. Coronal view above in schematic form clarifies the anatomical relationships here.

See illustration on opposite page.

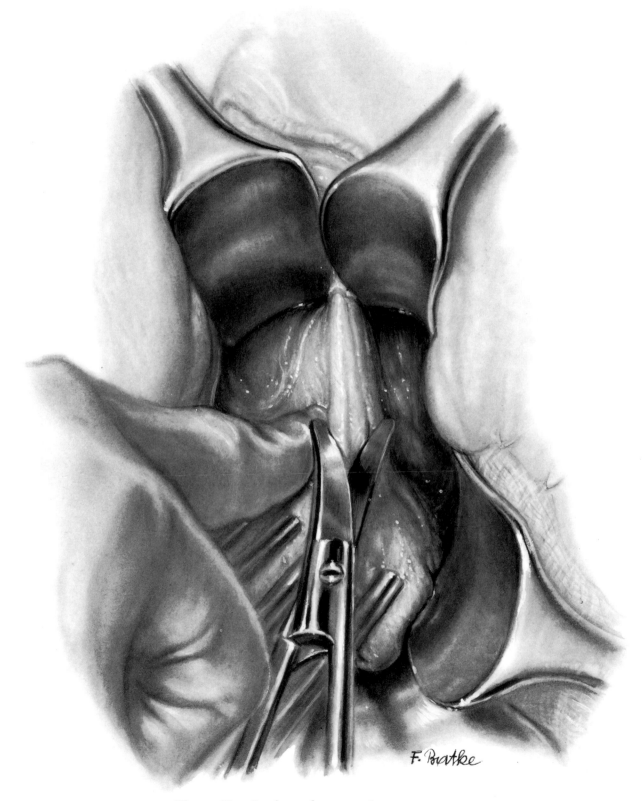

Figure 60. *See legend on opposite page.*

and a second somewhat wider one in the pararectal space. He pulls up and left with the anterior retractor and left and down with the posterior one. The operator depresses the left edge of the cervix down with his left index finger, stretching the bladder pillar in a sagittal direction. That part of the stretched bladder pillar near the cervix (vesicouterine ligament) is separated from the cervix anteriorly with several small scissors cuts (Fig. 60).

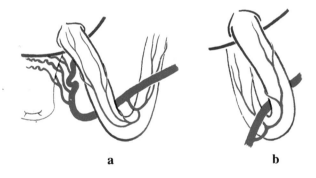

a   b

Figure 61.

Schauta-Amreich procedure. Placing the first ligature on the uterine vascular bundle. A portion of the bladder pillar has already been dissected from the cervix. The anterior spatulas stretch the remaining part of the bladder pillar. With proper dissection, the uterine vascular bundle appears at the edge of the cervix; the vessels are ligated here for the first time with a silk suture. The ligature is left long and pulled down to the right by the right assistant (who holds it together with the mouse-toothed clamps). Because the uterine artery crosses over the ureteral knee, downward traction on this vessel will displace the ureteral knee caudally to make it more accessible for mobilization. Relationships of the uterine artery and the ureteric artery in situ (a) and after lateral displacement of the ureter (b) are shown above in the schematic diagrams.

See illustration on opposite page.

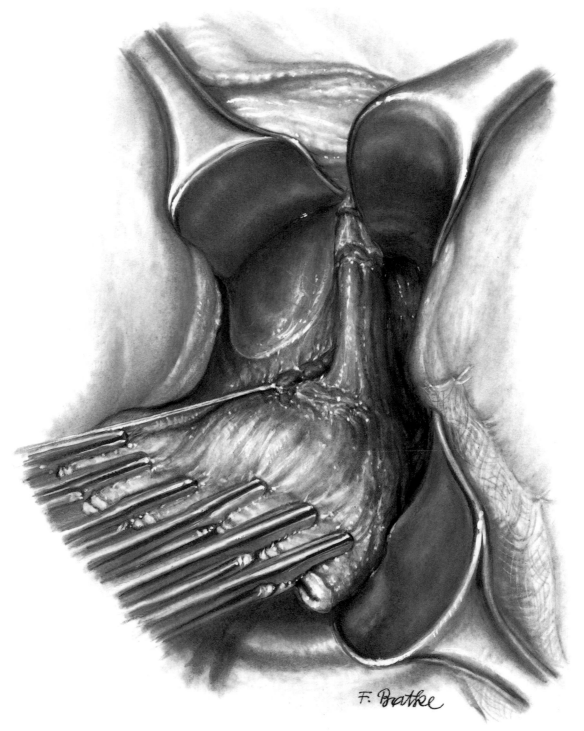

Figure 61. *See legend on opposite page.*

Following the separation of the caudal aspects of the bladder pillar, one approaches the ureteral knee coursing, as aforementioned, in the cranial part of the bladder pillar. It is not advisable to separate the bladder pillar from the cervix further at this time. Moreover, now the uterine vascular bundle (uterine artery and vein) can be found at the lateral margin of the cervix medially to the ureteral knee. The vessels are ligated by a silk suture applied around the bundle with a Deschamps aneurysm needle; the suture ends are left long for purposes of downward traction (Fig. 61).

Because the uterine vascular bundle always crosses over the ureteral knee, the ureter is dislocated somewhat downward by traction on the uterine ligature. Thus, the ureter can be located easily by renewed palpation to reconfirm its exact course in the bladder pillar. Having done this, one can now further divide the bladder pillar

Figure 62.

Schauta-Amreich procedure. Further separation of the bladder pillar from the cervix. By tilting the anterior speculum up, the remaining part of the bladder pillar is put on stretch so that the ureter can be palpated at the anterior edge of this sagitally oriented tissue layer. The freed uterine vascular bundle is religated cephalad to the first suture; the end is left long and pulled down to the right, further displacing the ureteral knee caudally. The surgeon carefully renews the division of the bladder pillar fibers with small scissor incisions near the cervix.

See illustration on opposite page.

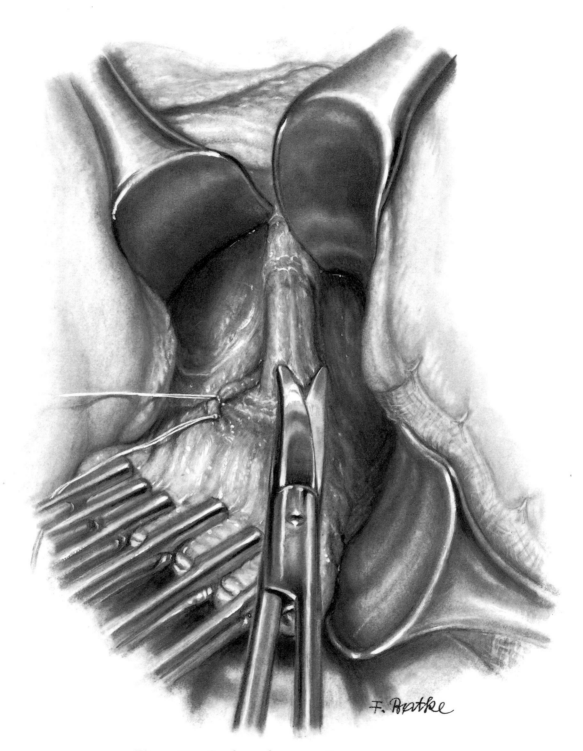

Figure 62.   *See legend on opposite page.*

fibers caudad to the ureteral knee, separating the pillar from the wall of the cervix (Fig. 62). The freed uterine vascular bundle is now tied off in a stepwise fashion moving progressively upward with successive silk suture-ligatures. After dividing these bladder pillar fibers, the exposed ureteral knee can be advanced laterally and slightly cephalad with the closed curved scissors. This maneuver further exposes the uterine vessels that are situated medially to the ureter; these vessels can be religated higher up at this point.

Where the bladder pillar is especially thickened, it is necessary to ligate doubly and divide the tissue fibers that lie laterally to the

1. traction on ureteric vessel bundle
2. uterine vasculature
3. ureter

1. ureteric artery
2. uterine artery
3. ureter

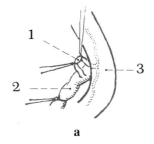

a

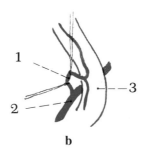

b

Figure 63.

Schauta-Amreich procedure. Opening the ureteral canal and ligating the ureteric artery. The remainder of the bladder pillar is stretched by vigorously tilting the anterior spatula. The medial aspects of the bladder pillar are completely separated from the cervix. The ureteral canal is opened and the ureteral knee is mobilized. The lateral remnants of the bladder pillar are yet to be dissected along the line indicated. The uterine vascular bundle is again ligated medially to the ureteral knee. The ureteric artery, originating from the uterine artery and coursing to the ureter, is doubly ligated, as shown above.

See illustration on opposite page.

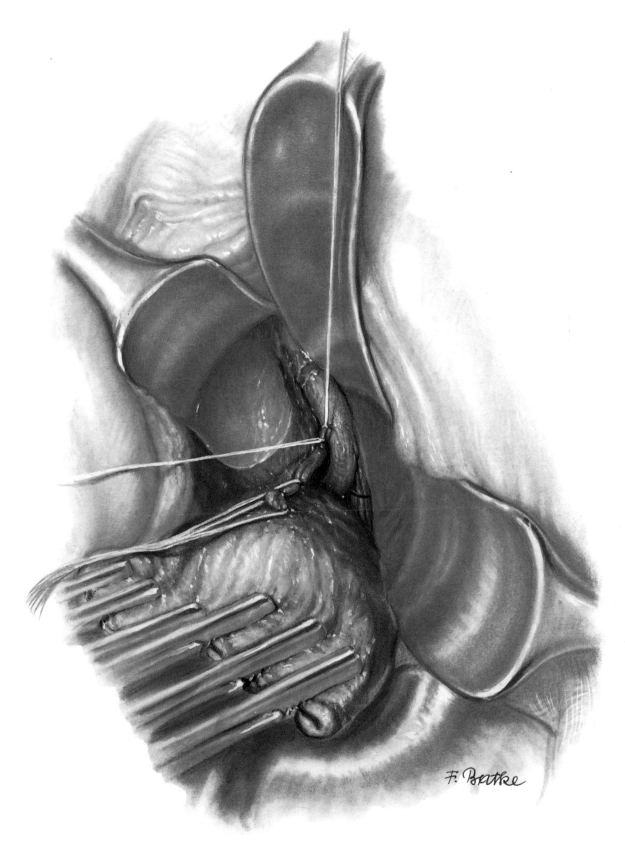

Figure 63.   *See legend on opposite page.*

ureteral knee. Thus, the ureteral knee that has already been freed medially, can be lifted upward somewhat with the closed dissecting scissors. Gradually, one exposes the stretched ureteric artery medially to the ureteral knee. This small branch of the uterine artery coursing to the ureter is doubly tied and divided (Fig. 63), thereby permitting one to elevate the ureteral knee still further (Fig. 64). At last it becomes possible to ligate the uterine vascular bundle twice very close to the pelvic sidewall (Fig. 65) and to resect it distally* to both ligatures (Fig. 66). The uterine ties that had been placed near the cervix are cut. The ureter is now completely mobilized (Fig. 67) and is easily elevated far up with the anterior spatula. This maneu-

*For purposes of clarifying orientation and direction, the authors have used the term distal here and elsewhere when referring to a site furthest away from the source of blood supply rather than the usual concept with regard to sites distant from the center or median line. The resection site here, for example, is mediad to the ties, albeit distal to the heart. — Ed.

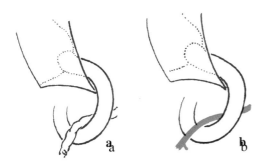

Figure 64.

Schauta-Amreich procedure. Displacement of the ureteral knee. The ureteric artery is divided. The uterine vessel bundle has been ligated several times and the uppermost suture end left long for traction. The surgeon pushes the mobilized ureteral knee further upward with the closed dissecting scissors, exposing more of the uterine vascular bundle that can now be ligated still higher. Exposure of the uterine vascular bundle (a) and of the uterine artery itself (b) is shown in the schematic figures above as it is accomplished in this step of the procedure.

See illustration on opposite page.

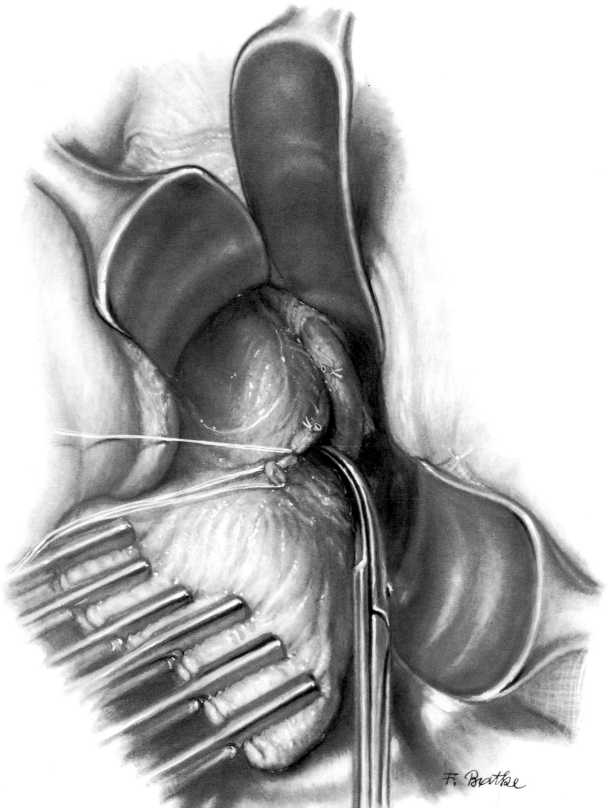

Figure 64.   *See legend on opposite page.*

ver, done by the assistant on the left, is of great importance in preparing for succeeding steps of the operation. A small gauze strip is temporarily placed in the paravesical space to control oozing of blood.

Technical Problems

1. If the bladder pillar is insufficiently stretched because the pressures on the retractors are incorrect, palpation of the ureteral knee is made more difficult and it becomes possible to injure the ureter during dissection of the caudal part of the bladder pillar.

2. When the fibers of the bladder pillar are dissected too close to the bladder, there may be danger to the ureter as well.

3. Should the bladder pillar be divided too near the cervix, massive hemorrhage from the uterine vessels may ensue.

4. In the event of insufficient dissection of the bladder pillar, freeing the ureteral knee becomes very difficult.

Figure 65.

Schauta-Amreich procedure. Final cephalad ligation of the uterine vessels. The left ureter is mobilized far up and laterally, being pushed cranially with the anterior spatula held by the left assistant. The anterior spatula of the right assistant elevates the bladder. Once again the uterine vascular bundle is doubly ligated up high.

See illustration on opposite page.

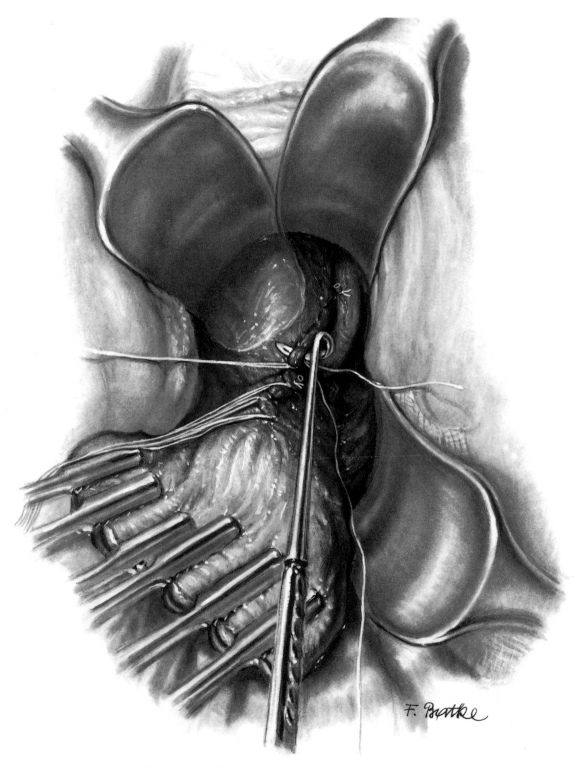

Figure 65.   *See legend on opposite page.*

5. When a cystocele coexists, the bladder may extend far down between the bladder pillars. It must first be carefully separated from the cervix and advanced before the uterine vessel bundle can be ligated up high. Otherwise, bladder tissue may be incorporated in the uterine ligature.

6. In the course of the sharp division of the bladder pillar from the cervix, the assistants must be sure to hold the vaginal spatula retractors very still, because every positional change produces a change in the location of the ureter within the bladder pillar.

7. If the right-side assistant does not apply sufficient continuous traction to the right and downward on the uppermost uterine vascular ligature, the ureteral knee in the bladder pillar is inadequately displaced caudally. Thus, the ureteral knee remains high up out of reach and is thereby more difficult to mobilize.

8. During the high ligation of the uterine vascular bundle, especially if some bleeding is occurring from it, that portion of the ureter near the bladder (the juxtavesical segment) may be drawn into the ligature.

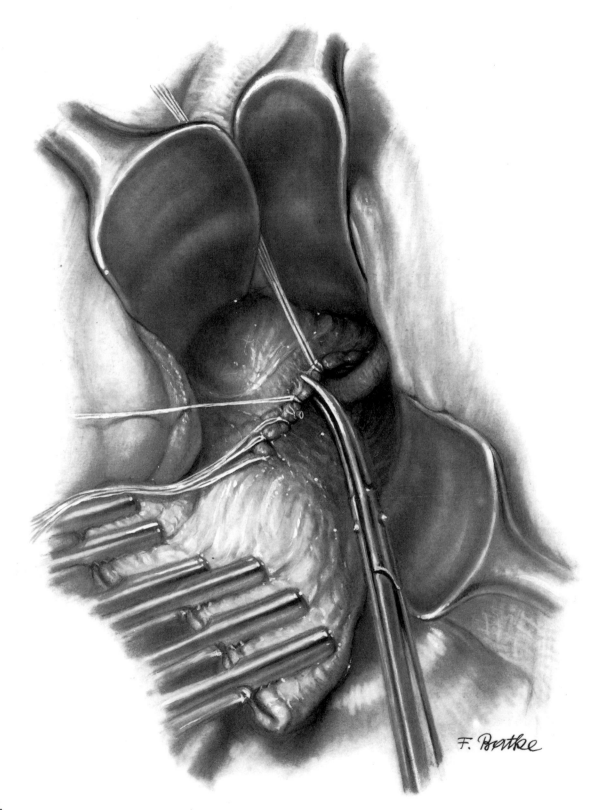

Figure 66.

Schauta-Amreich procedure. Division of the uterine vascular bundle. After high double ligation, the uterine vessels are divided with scissors distally to the uppermost ligature.

9. The left-side assistant can inadvertently tear veins located at the pelvic wall by excessive pressure applied to the spatulas in the paravesical and pararectal spaces. Tying these veins can create great difficulties.

The anatomy of these structures is detailed in the foregoing sections on ureter (see p. 42), pelvic connective tissue (see p. 58) and connective tissue spaces (see p. 64).

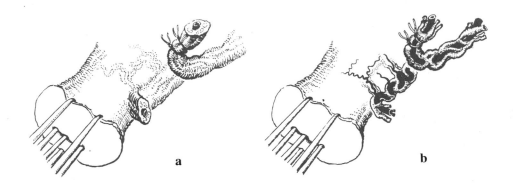

a   b

Figure 67.

Schauta-Amreich procedure. Mobilization of the freed left ureter after division of the uterine vessels. At the left edge of the cervix are the four uterine ligatures displayed by use of a wide spatula. Additionally, one can recognize the tongue-shaped peritoneal reflection reaching down the anterior uterine surface. The uterine vessels have been divided so that the ureteral knee is now no longer fixed. The ureter can be still further displaced upward by anterior spatula pressure applied by the left assistant. Medially to the freely mobilized ureteral knee, the cranial portion of the uterine vascular stump is visible. The schematics above demonstrate (a) the severed uterine vascular bundle and its contents (b), including the uterine artery and venous plexus.

See illustration on opposite page.

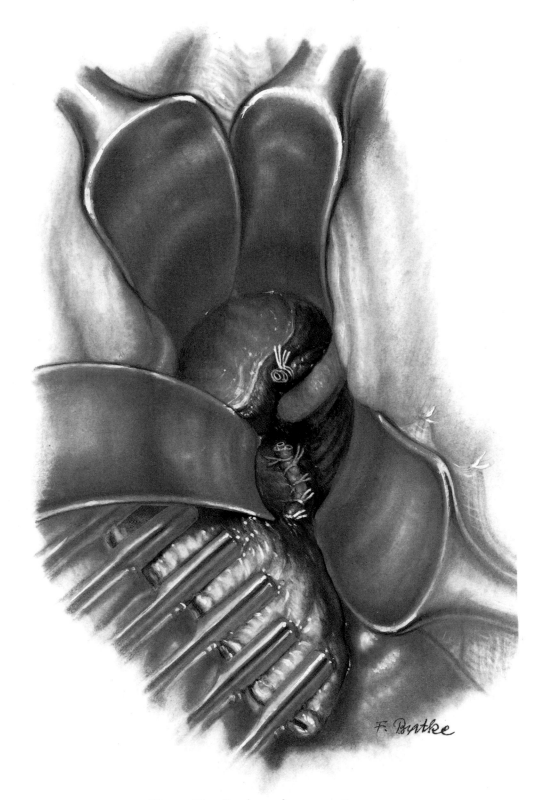

Figure 67. *See legend on opposite page.*

PREPARATION OF THE RIGHT PARA-SPACES

Opening the Right Paravesical Space

The right paravesical space must first be dissected in order to reach the lateral side of the right bladder pillar and expose it in its sagittal course. The approach is analogous to that which has been described for the left side.

Technique

The assistant on the left pulls the uterus to the left and down by the vaginal cuff; by means of an anterior spatula placed in the vesicocervical space he also lifts up on the bladder. The right assistant retracts the labia with an anterolateral spatula placed outside the vaginal wound edge. The surgeon applies two toothed clamps at the right mucosal margin of the vaginal circumcision wound, one up at the level of the paravesical space and the other further down at the pararectal space. He then pulls the upper clamp towards himself while the right assistant retracts the lower one downward.

The operator then opens the right paravesical space with a pair of curved dissecting scissors by incising at the level of the upper vaginal clamp just medially to the vaginal wall in between the vaginal fascia and the vesical fascia (Fig. 68). This entry into the right paravesical space is enlarged with the index finger until the entire paravesical space has been exposed. The right-side assistant now inserts an anterolateral spatula into this space and pushes the vaginal wall up and to the right. Additionally, with a posterolateral spatula, he depresses the rectum that is protruding into the pararectal space. The clamps are removed from the vaginal wound edges.

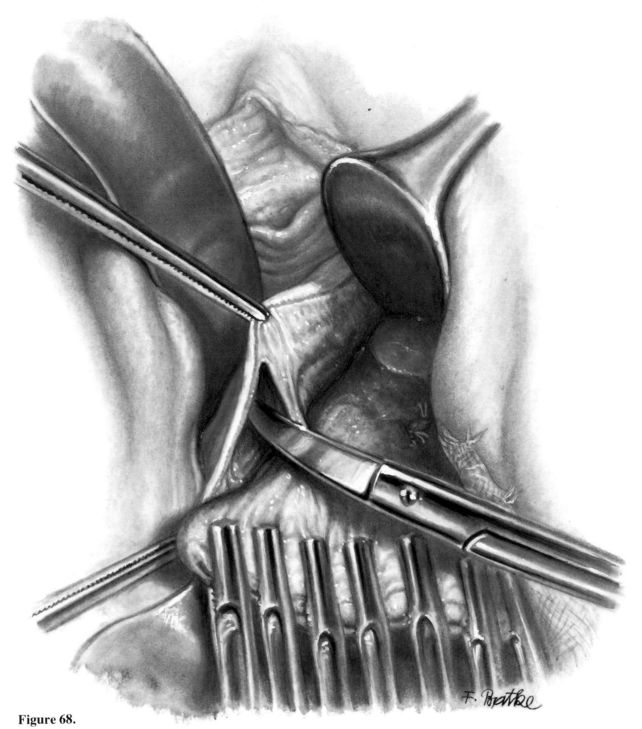

Figure 68.

Schauta-Amreich procedure. Opening the right paravesical space. The left assistant pushes the bladder up to the left with an anterior spatula inserted in the vesicocervical space (the anterior peritoneal reflection is seen); in addition, he pulls the mouse-toothed clamps attached to the vaginal cuff downward and to the left. The right labia are displaced to the right with an anterolateral spatula held in the right assistant's left hand. The surgeon places double-toothed claw tenacula on the circumcised vaginal wall at the level of the paravesical and the pararectal spaces so that the vaginal wound edge can be stretched here. He pulls the vaginal edge forward with the anterior paravesical tenaculum; the posterior pararectal tenaculum is held by the right assistant's right hand. The operator dissects between the vaginal incision edge and the right bladder pillar with the scissors to open the right paravesical space.

Correct and complete exposure of the right paravesical space sometimes presents more difficulties even to an experienced vaginal surgeon than mobilization of the ureters (see p. 112).

Technical Problems

1. The sharp dissection required for opening the paravesical space must be carried out just under the vaginal fascia. If one incises somewhat more medially, bladder injury can occur easily.

2. The scissors may be directed incorrectly during the opening into the space. If the vaginal circumcision had been done relatively close to the portio so that only a small amount of vagina was circumcised for later removal, the closed tip of the scissors for opening the paravesical space must be directed laterally in order to be certain that it will proceed laterally to the right bladder pillar. On the other hand, if plenty of vaginal canal is being removed (that is, the circumcision was carried out far down from the portio), the tip of the dissecting scissors should proceed instead directly upward into the paravesical space, much more parallel with the pelvic wall. If it were to be directed laterally it might reach the obturator fascia and cause injury to the pelvic wall veins.

3. After the paravesical space has been opened, if the scissors tip is advanced too far into the space, the veins at the pelvic wall or the bladder can be damaged. Complete exposure of the opened paravesical space is best done bluntly by digital dissection.

4. If one should not open the space widely enough, one finds that it will not be possible subsequently to expose the outer surface of the right bladder pillar completely. This deficiency will make dissection of the ureter considerably more difficult.

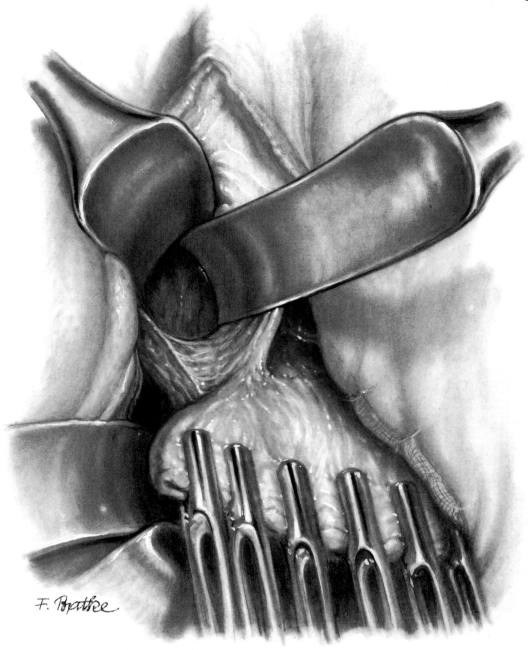

F. Bathe

Figure 69.

Schauta-Amreich procedure. Exposing the right horizontal pelvic fascia. The right paravesical space is opened and spread by two anterior spatulas inserted into it. The left assistant advances the long, narrow spatula in this space medially to the right bladder pillar. The lateral wall of the paravesical space is pushed cranially with the spatula held by the right assistant. The right assistant pushes the rectum down with a posterolateral spatula in the pararectal space. The horizontal pelvic fascia is recognized as the layer separating the paravesical and pararectal spaces.

DISSECTION OF THE RIGHT HORIZONTAL PELVIC FASCIA

The horizontal pelvic fascia represents the interfacing layer between the right paravesical space and the right pararectal space. It can be readily exposed if the left assistant places a very narrow spatula into the right paravesical space and pushes the bladder pillar somewhat medially while the right assistant retracts the right vaginal wall to the right with retractors inserted into both paraspaces (Fig. 69).

Technique

The pliable connective tissue layer becomes horizontal when pressure is applied on the spatulas as described. The fascia is doubly clamped (Fig. 70) and divided between the clamps. The clamps are then replaced by catgut sutures. After the horizontal pelvic fascia has been cut, the right paravesical space is united with the right pararectal space. In this way the spaces lateral to the bladder pillar and the rectum are completely prepared.

Technical Problems

1. If the clamps are applied too high up the pelvic wall on the horizontal pelvic fascia, the blood vessels at the pelvic wall can be injured by the lateral clamp, and the ureter coursing in the bladder pillar can be injured by the medial clamp.

2. In suturing the stump held in the correctly placed medial clamp, one must not insert the needle too deeply into the bladder pillar because the ureter can be tied off as a result.

3. Incomplete union of the right paravesical space with the pararectal space will risk later difficulty by virtue of the thickened tissue that will be encountered while attempting to dissect the right ureteral knee free. This tissue courses in a craniocaudal direction and may be part of the descended bladder or the levator. It is essential that any connective tissue found laterally to the ureteral knee must be moved aside or divided in order to achieve complete mobilization; if this is not done, it is possible to injure the bladder here.

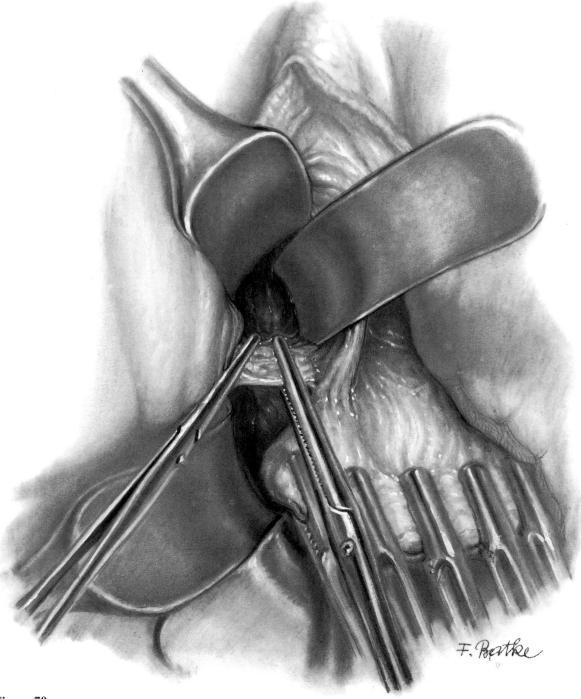

Figure 70.

Schauta-Amreich procedure. Uniting the paravesical and pararectal spaces. The horizontal fascia is positioned by appropriate spatula pressures. It is clamped with two long, straight clamps and divided between them.

EXPOSURE OF THE RIGHT URETER

Dissection of the ureter on the right is done in an analogous manner to that on the left. The left-side assistant pulls the uterus down and to the left, simultaneously elevating the bladder with an anterior spatula in the vesicocervical space. The bladder pillar is thereby stretched in a sagittal plane (Fig. 71). The assistant on the right retracts the vaginal wall upward and to the right with a spatula placed anterolaterally in the right paravesical space, while with another somewhat wider spatula in the right pararectal space he

Figure 71.

Schauta-Amreich procedure. Presentation of the right bladder pillar. The right horizontal pelvic fascia is divided and the clamps are replaced by catgut sutures, uniting the paravesical and pararectal spaces. The left assistant elevates the bladder with a spatula in the vesicocervical space, medially to the right bladder pillar, and pulls the vaginal cuff down to the left. At the anterior uterine wall, one can see the tongue-like peritoneal reflection. Laterally to the bladder pillar, the right assistant pushes the vaginal incision edge upward to the right with a narrow anterolateral spatula in the paravesical space, while holding back the rectum with a somewhat wider posterolateral spatula in the pararectal space. The right bladder pillar is taut and can be further stretched by tilting the anterior spatula.

See illustration on opposite page.

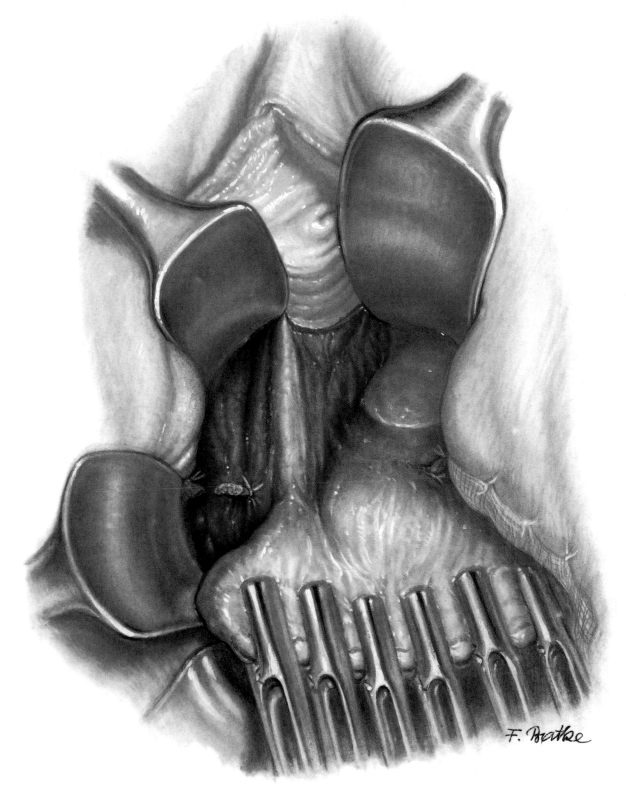

Figure 71. *See legend on opposite page.*

pulls down and to the right. The surgeon locates the ureteral knee by palpation (Fig. 72), dividing the caudal part of the bladder pillar close to the cervix (Fig. 73). Next, he ties off the uterine vascular bundle with a series of stepwise ligatures. He advances progressively up along the vascular pedicle with each suture, pushing the bladder pillar further and further from the cervix, partially by incising it and partially by blunt pressure, until the ureteral knee is freed in front. The left assistant applies traction downward on the uppermost uterine ligature so that the ureteral knee is displaced caudally for purposes of easier dissection (Fig. 74).

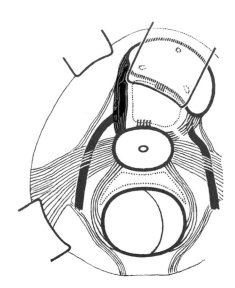

Figure 72.

Schauta-Amreich procedure. Palpating the right ureter in the bladder pillar. The right bladder pillar is positioned by means of appropriate spatula pressures and is recognizable as a connective tissue layer in the sagittal plane. The surgeon determines the course of the ureteral knee by palpation with his second and third fingers by taking hold of the bladder pillar in a scissor-like grip. The severed left vesicouterine ligament and stretched intact right vesicouterine ligament are shown above with their relations to the ureters illustrated.

See illustration on opposite page.

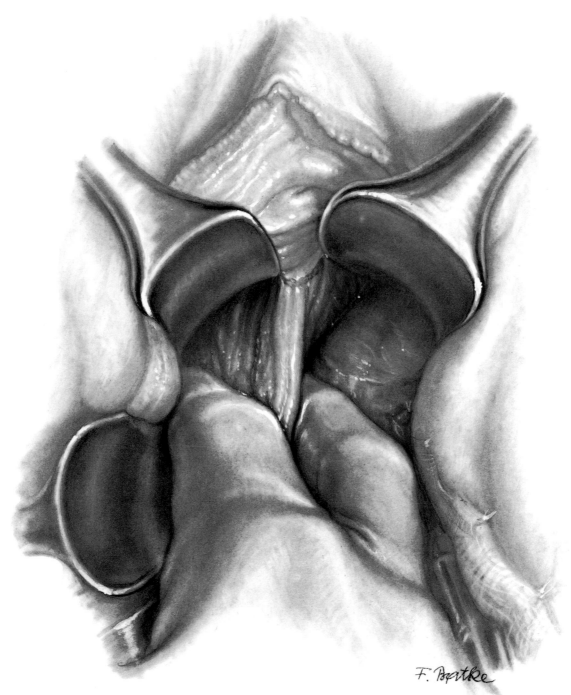

Figure 72.   *See legend on opposite page.*

In cases where there is much vaginal or bladder descensus the bladder edge must be dissected off the ureteral knee both laterally and medially and advanced upward before proceeding (Figs. 75 and 76). After the ureter has been mobilized further, the uterine vessels are doubly ligated high up and divided (Fig. 77). This step concludes the bilateral ureteral dissection. Tamponade of the right paravesical space is now accomplished by means of a small gauze strip to staunch any bleeding.

(Text continued on page 150)

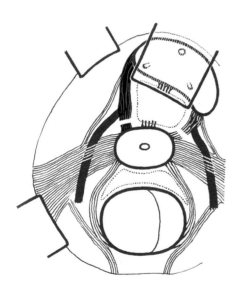

Figure 73.

Schauta-Amreich procedure. Dividing the right bladder pillar at the cervix. The assistants stretch the bladder pillar by exerting upward pressure on the spatulas while simultaneously tilting them. Additionally, the right assistant holds back the rectum with his posterolateral spatula. The surgeon depresses the cervix with his left index finger and incises the bladder pillar at its base close to the edge of the cervix. The situation at this point, with both vesicouterine ligaments severed, is shown schematically above.

See illustration on opposite page.

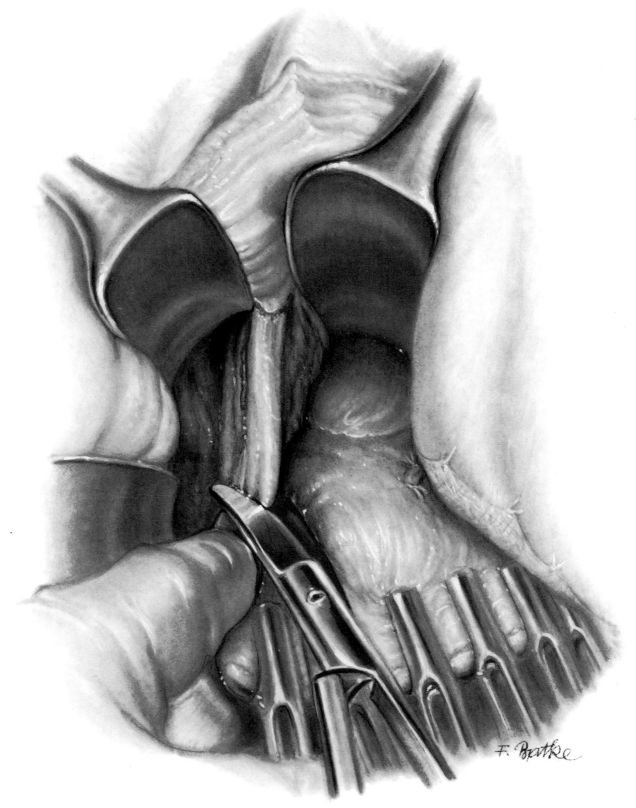

Figure 73.   *See legend on opposite page.*

Figure 74.

Schauta-Amreich procedure. Dissection of the lateral bladder pole from the cervix. The right vaginal wall is pushed laterally by the right assistant with two lateral spatulas. The bladder base is lifted toward the symphysis by the left assistant's anterior spatula. The right bladder pillar is partially separated from the cervix. The uterine vascular bundle is ligated and the suture is left long for downward traction to the left by the left assistant who pulls it together with the mouse-toothed clamps which are attached to the vaginal cuff. Medially to the exposed ureter is the lateral descending bladder margin, here adherent somewhat to the cervix by virtue of previous inflammation. The operator raises the fixed bladder edge with toothed forceps. The lateral bladder pole is now placed on stretch and can be divided close to the cervix with scissors.

See illustration on opposite page.

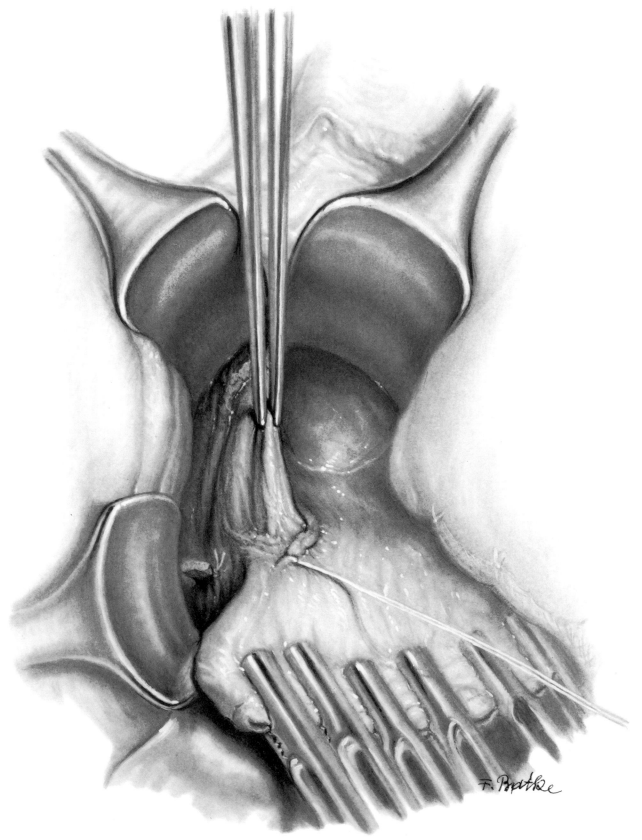

Figure 74.   *See legend on opposite page.*

Figure 75.

Schauta-Amreich procedure. Ligating the lateral aspects of the bladder pillar. The remaining portion of the bladder pillar is stretched by appropriate spatula pressure. The ureter is extensively mobilized on its medial side. The uterine vascular bundle has already been ligated three times previously; the uppermost of these ligatures is pulled downward to the left. Those fibers of the thickened bladder pillar which course laterally to the ureter can be doubly ligated and divided between the sutures (only after this step can the ureteral knee be properly mobilized). The points of the closed scissors are in the opened ureteral canal, elevating the ureteral knee in order to relocate it out of the line of incision.

See illustration on opposite page.

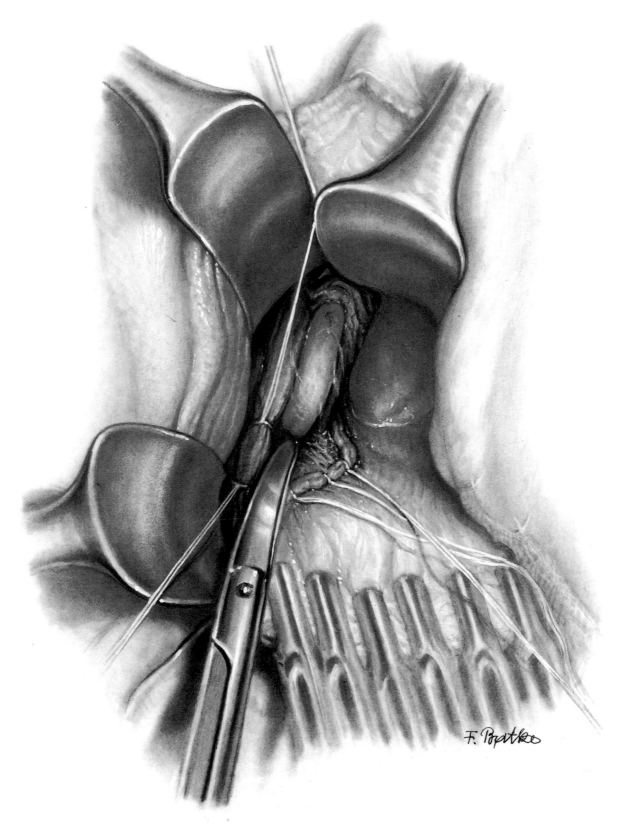

Figure 75.   *See legend on opposite page.*

Figure 76.

Schauta-Amreich procedure. Further separation of the bladder pillar from the cervix. The lateral aspects of the bladder pillar have been ligated and dissected; the uterine vessels have been ligated three times. By tilting and forcefully elevating the anterior spatulas, the remaining fibers of the bladder pillar medially to the ureter are stretched; they are dissected close to the cervix with scissors. In order to avoid injuring the ureter, the curved tips of the scissors are pointed toward the cervix during the dissection.

See illustration on opposite page.

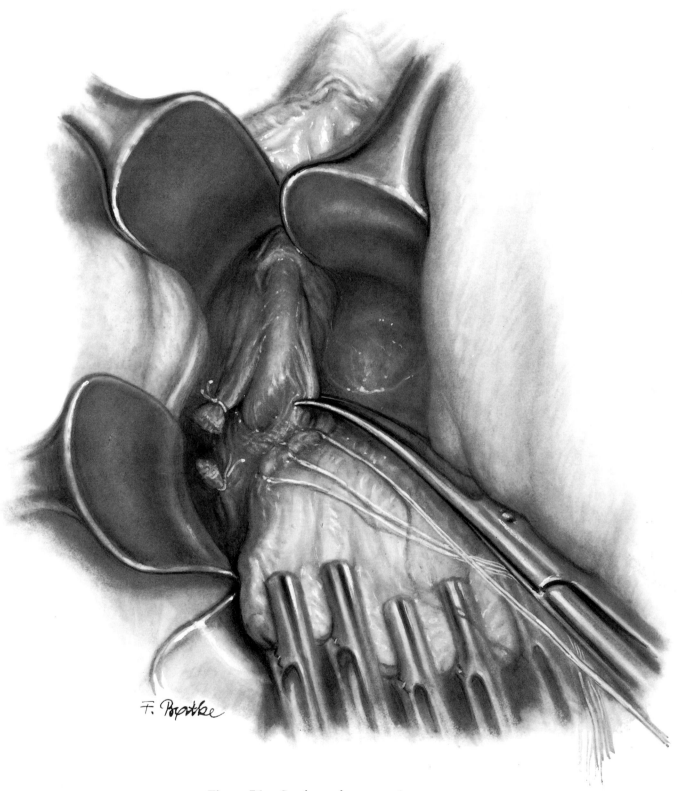

Figure 76.   *See legend on opposite page.*

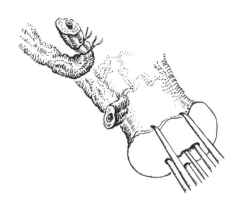

Figure 77.

Schauta-Amreich procedure. Appearance of the operative site after division of the uterine vascular bundle. The right ureter is freely mobilized. After the multiply ligated uterine vascular bundle is divided high up, it can be dislocated upward and laterally with a spatula. An anterior spatula elevates the bladder base. On the median aspect of the uterus, one can recognize the anterior peritoneal reflection. The severed ligatures of the uterine vessels, previously ligated in stepwise fashion, are visible at the lateral border of the cervix. Division of the uterine vessel bundle is shown in the diagram above.

See illustration on opposite page.

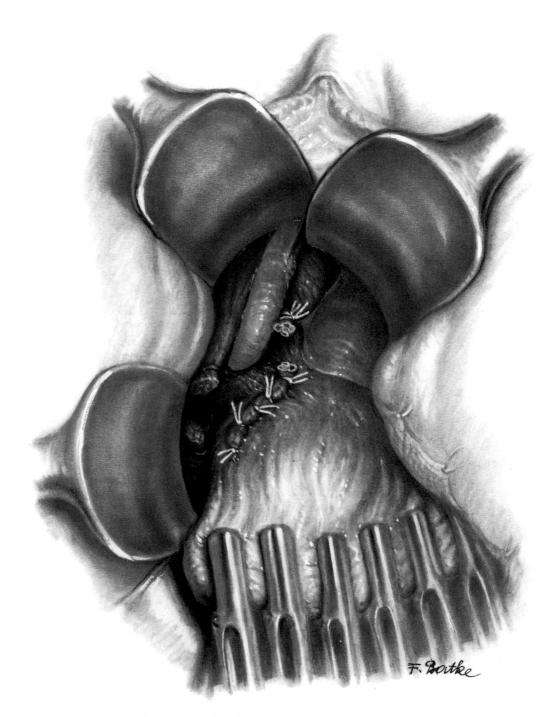

Figure 77.   *See legend on opposite page.*

OPENING THE PERITONEAL CULDESAC

Technique

The right assistant pulls the uterus up toward the symphysis pubis with his left hand by traction on the series of mouse-toothed clamps; he also depresses the rectum, which is usually ballooning forward, with the spatula in the right pararectal space. The left assistant inserts another spatula in the right pararectal space; this he holds in his right hand while he simultaneously grasps the posterior self-retaining vaginal retractor with his left hand, applying downward pressure on the rectum with both (Fig. 78). The surgeon pushes the rectum caudally in the midline with dissecting scissors held slightly opened and pointed upward (or using a gauze sponge for dissection) until the peritoneal culdesac reflection (Douglas fold, plica rectouterina) becomes readily accessible. He grasps the peritoneal edge with toothed tissue forceps and divides it above the forceps with a single cut of the scissors (Fig. 79). A silk tie is secured in the midline at the posterior peritoneal wound edge and left long for purposes of downward traction on the posterior peritoneum.

Technical Problems

1. If the rectum is dissected off the posterior wall too far laterally, the stretched tissue fibers located at the sides will be di-

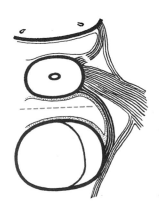

Figure 78.

Schauta-Amreich procedure. Preparation of the operative field for opening the culdesac of Douglas. The vaginal cuff with its attached mouse-toothed clamps is lifted toward the symphysis by the right assistant's left hand. The left assistant's left hand depresses the self-retaining posterior retractor toward the sacrum. Both assistants retract the vagina and rectum aside with lateral spatulas. The anteriorly ballooning peritoneum of the space of Douglas is recognized. The diagram above shows the culdesac of Douglas situated between cervix and rectum.

See illustration on opposite page.

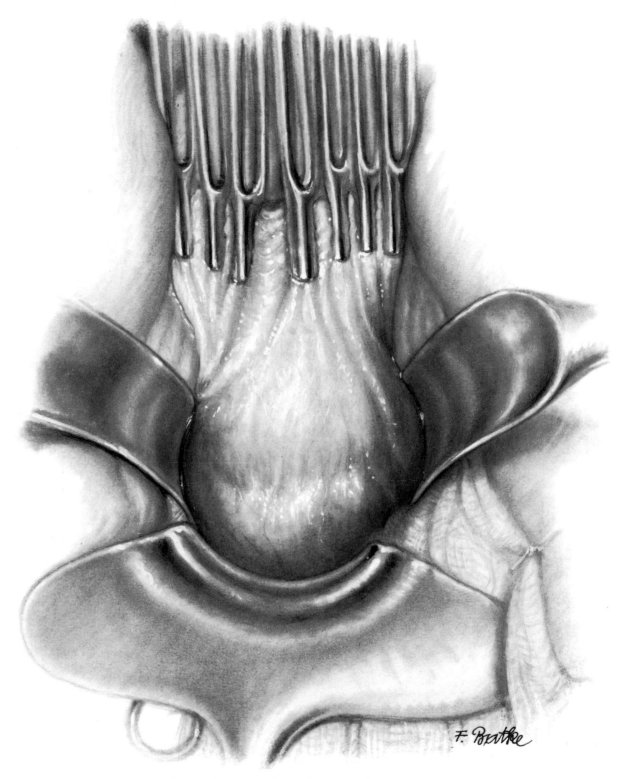

Figure 78. *See legend on opposite page.*

vided. These fibers are part of the rectal pillar, constituting the uterosacral ligaments that should not be dissected close to the posterior cervix at this time, but, instead, close to the rectum later in the procedure.

2. The peritoneal culdesac reflection may be sought too near the cervix by virtue of fear concerning injury to the rectum. This will cause the operator to dissect the posterior peritoneum further and further away from the posterior wall of the cervix. He will be working in a poor plane and he will therefore not be able to locate the abdominal cavity. Under these circumstances, it is advisable to pull the incorrectly dissected tissues upward with a toothed clamp and to incise caudally to the clamp. Then the posterior peritoneal reflection can be opened without risk, provided there are no adhesions in the culdesac.

3. It is sometimes not feasible to prepare the peritoneal reflection clearly, if at all. If the operator should try to open it with a single incision under these suboptimal conditions, he is embarking on a dangerous course that is preferably avoided, because it may seriously injure the rectum or a loop of small intestine. Ordinarily, dissection in the correct layer will permit clear definition of the culdesac and make it easy to open. One should assume that adhesions are present if the peritoneum cannot be readily found; here it is better not to try to open the culdesac at this time, but to await a better view of the situation in the Douglas space later, after the vesicouterine fold has been opened and the uterus has been rolled anteriorly.

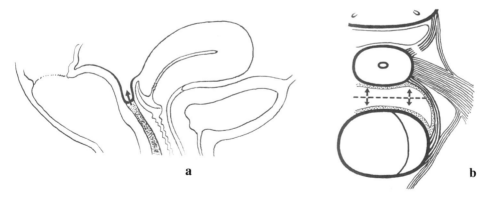

a   b

Figure 79.

Schauta-Amreich procedure. Opening the peritoneum. The peritoneum of the space of Douglas is grasped in the midline with toothed forceps and it is opened cephalad to this site with a transverse scissors incision. During this step, the curved tips of the scissors should point upward to the posterior wall of the cervix. Schematic representations of culdesac relationships are shown in sagittal (a) and coronal (b) sections above.

See illustration on opposite page.

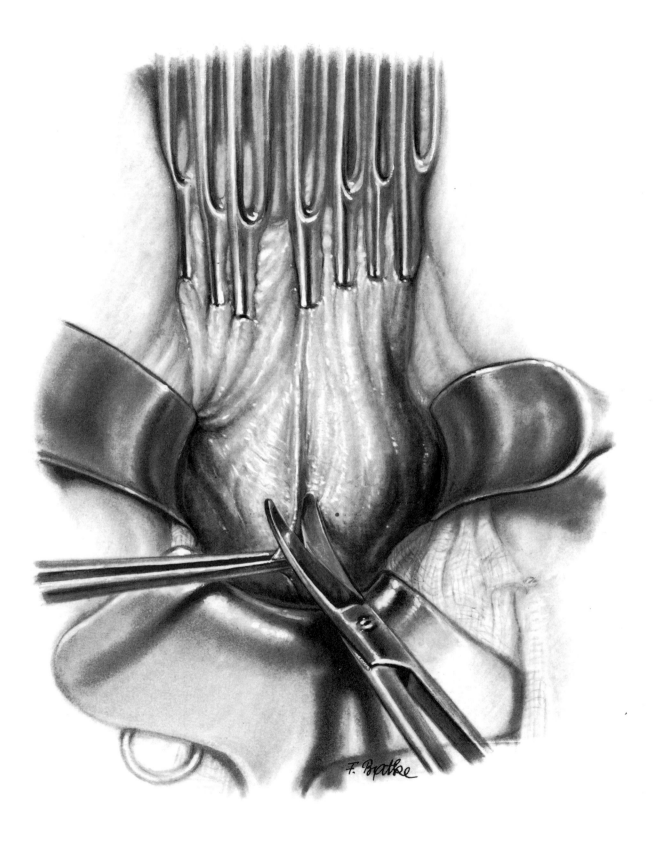

Figure 79.   *See legend on opposite page.*

DIVISION OF THE RECTAL PILLARS

Positioning the Rectal Pillar

The gauze sponges tamponading the paravesical spaces are removed. A long gauze strip is inserted into the culdesac of Douglas, ostensibly to keep intestinal loops out of the field. The gauze is pushed up by the right-side assistant using a broad right-angled retractor that simultaneously also displaces the bowel. In addition, the right assistant pulls the uterus up toward the symphysis by means of traction on the vaginal cuff. This stretches the rectal pillars so that they become sagittally oriented, coursing upward from the sides of rectum to the cardinal ligaments.

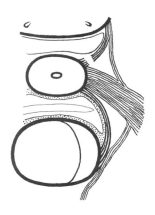

Figure 80.

Schauta-Amreich procedure. Preparing the operative field for dissection of the left bladder pillar. The space of Douglas is opened widely and a silk traction suture is placed at the posterior peritoneal edge. The bowel is packed back with a large intraperitoneal gauze strip, held in place by a wide, right-angled retractor inserted in the pelvic cavity and lifted upward by the right hand of the right assistant; his left hand also elevates the mouse-toothed clamps on the vaginal cuff toward the symphysis. The left assistant lifts the ureter with a long, narrow anterolateral spatula and pushes back the rectum with a somewhat wider posterolateral one. The left rectal pillar (ligamentum rectouterinum) is thereby stretched so that it courses upward from the left lateral edge of the rectum to Mackinrodt's ligament. This tissue structure is located sagittally and is covered by peritoneum on its medial surface as shown diagrammatically above.

See illustration on opposite page.

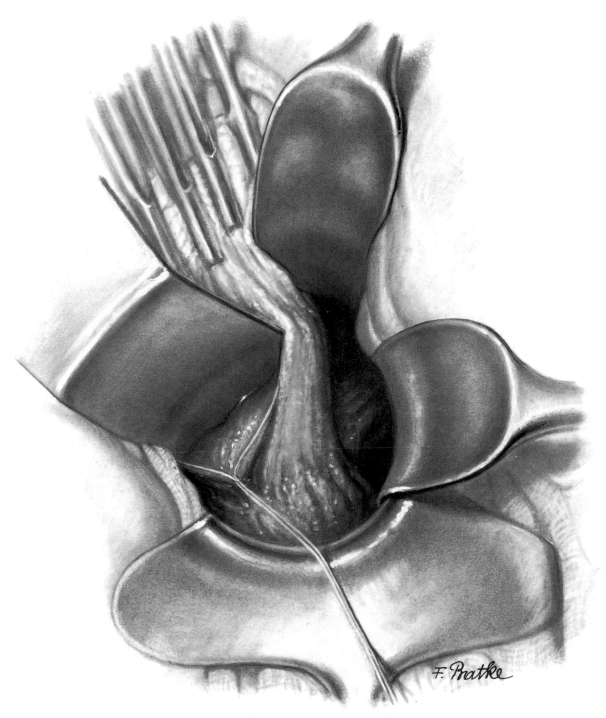

Figure 80.   *See legend on opposite page.*

Division of the Left Rectal Pillar

The right assistant pushes the bowel up and to the right with a wide right-angled retractor in his right hand, and pulls the mouse-toothed clamps on the vaginal stump in the same direction with his left hand. The left assistant advances the mobilized left ureter far cranially with a long narrow spatula placed in the left paravesical fossa and held in his right hand. The surgeon should assure himself by visual check that the left ureter has actually been relocated well out of the way. The left-side assistant's left hand applies caudal pressure on the lateral aspects of the rectum with a spatula placed in the left pararectal fossa. This stretches and clearly identifies the left rectal pillar (Fig. 80).

The surgeon undermines and bluntly loosens the peritoneum at the medial side of the left rectal pillar with closed scissors. He then incises the peritoneum at the base of the rectal pillar close to the rectum (Fig. 81), extending the incision until it reaches cranially to the entrance of the rectal pillar into the left Mackinrodt ligament. Next, he pushes the rectum toward the sacrum with a sponge forceps or a retractor inserted into the space of Douglas, displacing the rectal pillar that has just been freed from the peritoneum. The rectal pillar is therefore easily delineated and can be clamped close to the rectum (Fig. 82). Alternatively, the rectal pillar can be divided without clamping; however, the more cranial the incision here, the more likely it will traverse the rectal artery that courses in the rectal pillar. If cut, this vessel may retract during free dissection and the ensuing bleeding will be very difficult to control.

Figure 81.

Schauta-Amreich procedure. Incision of the peritoneum at the left rectal pillar. The peritoneum that adheres medially to the rectal pillar is dissected from it. An incision is made in the peritoneum at the base of the pillar along the left lateral edge of the rectum and extended upward.

See illustration on opposite page.

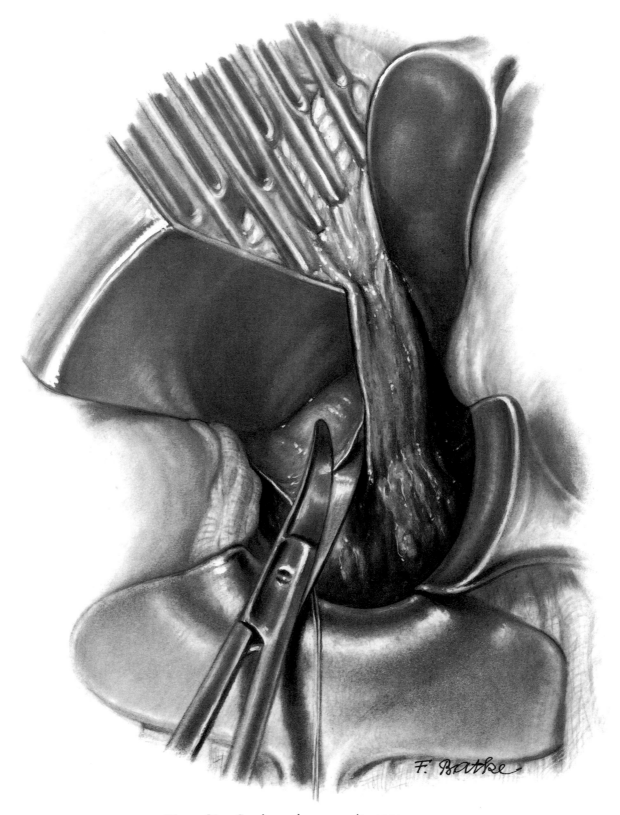

Figure 81.   *See legend on opposite page.*

Technical Problems

1. The peritoneum medially to the rectal pillar may be incised too far cranially, creating difficulties later when it becomes necessary to reperitonealize at this high level.

2. If the ureter is not adequately displaced with the spatula held by the left assistant during the division of the rectal pillar, ureteral damage is likely to result.

3. When the rectal pillar is separated too high cephalad, hemorrhage may occur from Mackinrodt's ligament.

4. Should the rectum balloon medially and not be sufficiently displaced caudally, rectal injury is possible as the rectal pillar is resected close to the rectum.

5. If the entire rectal pillar is boldly mobilized, hemorrhage can ensue from the medial hemorrhoidal artery.

Dissection of the Right Rectal Pillar

The bowel is guarded by a gauze pad inserted intraperitoneally and is retracted up to the left by the left-side assistant with a wide right-angled spatula held in his left hand. The vaginal cuff is pulled

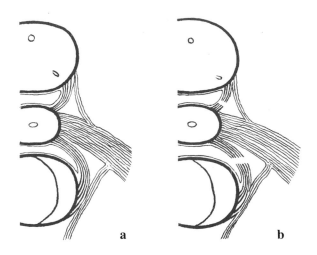

a   b

Figure 82.

Schauta-Amreich procedure. Clamping the left rectal pillar. The left rectal pillar is stretched in the sagittal plane. The base has been exposed by previous dissection of its medial peritoneal leaf; two long, straight clamps are applied here close to the rectum. The rectal pillar can be divided between these clamps. Schematically illustrated above are the anatomical relationships of the connective tissues before (a) and after (b) division of the vesicouterine and rectouterine ligaments.

See illustration on opposite page.

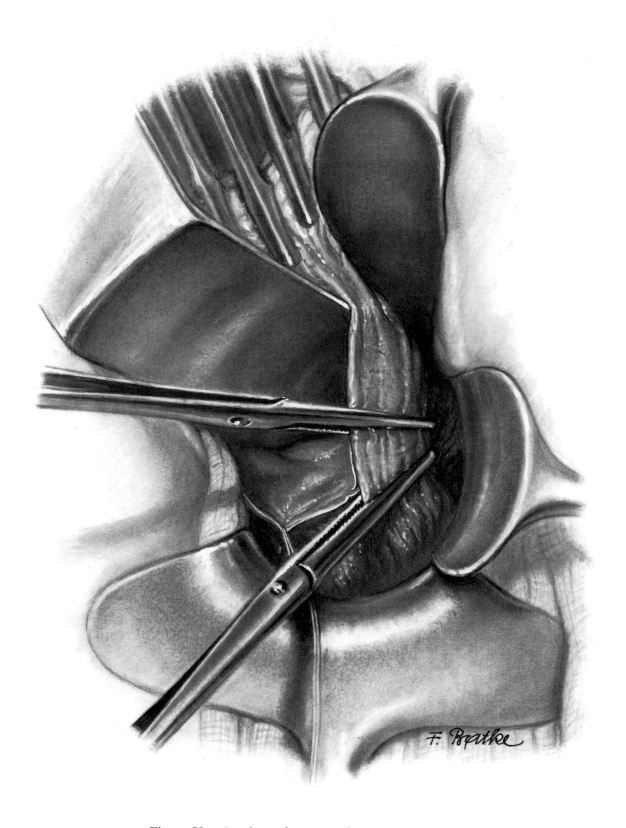

Figure 82. *See legend on opposite page.*

in the same direction with his right hand. The right assistant protects the ureter with a long spatula held in the left hand and inserted in the right paravesical space; the ureter is pushed upward in this manner. The assistant on the right also applies downward pressure on the rectum with a spatula placed in the right pararectal space, stretching the rectal pillar (Fig. 83). The surgeon then undermines and incises the peritoneum just as was done to the medial side of the right rectal pillar. Thus, he dissects the pillar and divides it between clamps close to the rectum.

Figure 83.

Schauta-Amreich procedure. Dissecting the rectum. The left assistant holds the bowel back with the wide right-angled retractor in his left hand and lifts the mouse-toothed clamps on the vaginal cuff toward the symphysis with his right hand. The right assistant elevates the ureter with a long spatula in the paravesical space and depresses the rectum with a spatula in the pararectal space. A silk traction suture is fastened to the posterior peritoneal cut edge. The right rectal pillar is thus prepared. The forward-ballooning rectum must be dissected somewhat more from its attachments to the outer aspects of the right rectal pillar so that it is not damaged when the pillar is divided. To accomplish this the surgeon depresses the anterior rectal wall with a sponge forceps inserted intraperitoneally while pushing the rectum toward the sacrum with slightly opened curved dissecting scissors (with tips pointing upward).

See illustration on opposite page.

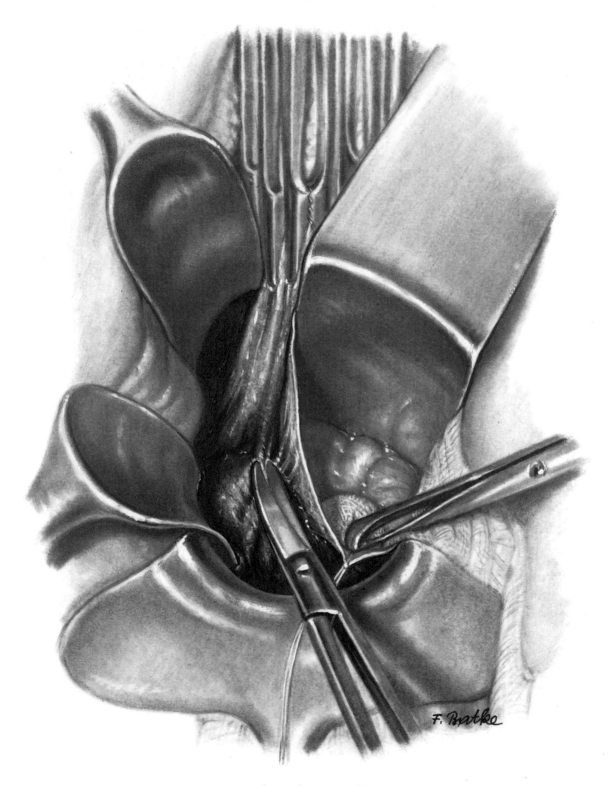

Figure 83. *See legend on opposite page.*

OPENING THE VESICOUTERINE PLICA

Technique

The uterus is retracted sacrally by the left assistant, who pulls down on the mouse-toothed clamps attached to the vaginal stump. The right assistant elevates the mobilized bladder toward the symphysis with an anterior spatula. The vesicouterine plica is easily recognized at the anterior surface of the uterus as a tongue of shiny peritoneal reflection. It is lifted slightly off the anterior uterus with a pair of curved tissue forceps and is opened distally with one cut of the scissors. A light silk ligature fixed to the peritoneal wound edge serves for traction (Fig. 84). The peritoneal opening is enlarged on both sides with scissors. The right assistant now enters the widely opened peritoneal space with the anterior retractor, pulling up on the anterior peritoneal edge and the bladder. The surgeon introduces a second long tamponade into the peritoneal opening for the purpose of preventing intestinal loops from prolapsing.

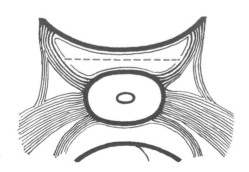

Figure 84.

Schauta-Amreich procedure. Opening the anterior peritoneum. The uterus is pulled downward by the left assistant. The right assistant elevates the bladder with a spatula in the vesicocervical space. The vagina is spread by two lateral spatulas and the plica vesicouterina of the peritoneum is opened. A silk traction suture is placed at the anterior peritoneal cut edge. Entrance into the peritoneal cavity anteriorly is shown above in schematic form.

See illustration on opposite page.

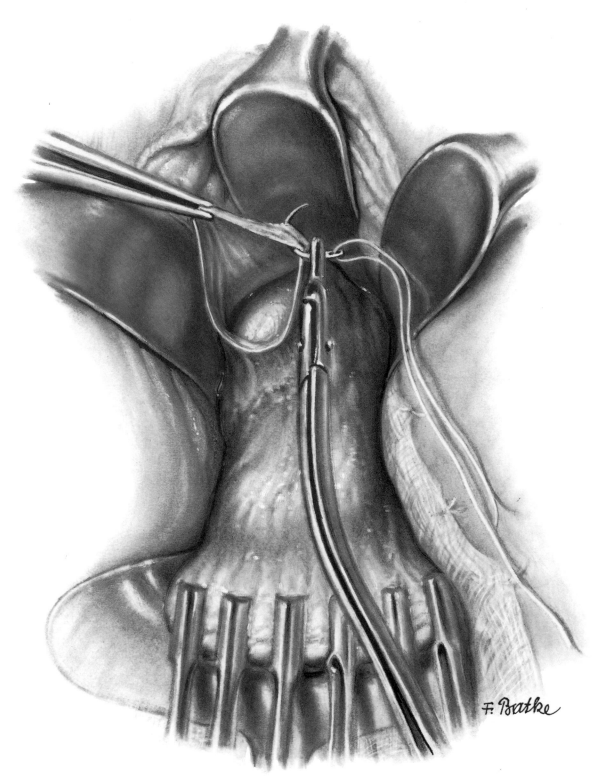

Figure 84. *See legend on opposite page.*

Technical Problems

1. If the silk used as a ligature at the anterior peritoneal edge is too heavy, the peritoneum may tear at the slightest pull. This is seen especially in obese patients whose peritoneum may be particularly thin and easily torn.

2. If the needle used to suture the anterior peritoneal wound edge is too large, the peritoneum will tear during manipulation of the needle in the limited room of the vesicouterine space. The suture pulls out as a consequence and the peritoneal edge retracts.

3. While tamponading the bowel, one must ensure that the anterior retractor has been inserted intraabdominally and that the anterior peritoneal wound edge is adequately supported. If the gauze pad is held too forcibly in place by the spatula, the silk traction suture at the anterior peritoneal edge will tear out or the peritoneum will tear laterally and far upward. This latter type of high peritoneal tear can be difficult to repair.

RESECTION OF THE ADNEXA (IN CONJUNCTION WITH THE UTERUS)

Anteversion of the Uterus

The bladder and loops of bowel are held back and advanced upward with a wide right-angled retractor inserted intraperitoneally by the right-side assistant. The surgeon grasps the uterine fundus with a double-toothed (claw) tenaculum placed close to the tubal junction, pulling the corpus uteri out of the peritoneal cavity. Tilting out the uterus can be simplified if the left assistant simultaneously pushes the vaginal vault toward the sacrum into the space of Douglas using the attached mouse-toothed clamps (Fig. 85).

Technical Problems

1. The claw tenaculum may not be applied high enough on the fundus of the uterus. Sometimes one has to "climb up" along the anterior wall of the corpus with several single-toothed tenacula before the claw forceps can be applied to the fundus.

2. When there are adhesions present between the uterus and the omentum, the intestine or the adnexa, such adhesions must first be carefully lysed, both sharply and bluntly, before the uterus can be rolled forward. Persistent adhesions prevent safe successful completion of this step in the procedure. The adhesions must always be

divided under direct vision, preferably with small bites of the dissection scissors.

Division of the Right Infundibulopelvic and Round Ligaments

The left-side assistant retracts the bladder and the bowel up and to the left with a right-angled spatula placed intraperitoneally while pulling the tenaculum on the fundus to the left along with the clamps on the vaginal vault. The right assistant inserts another spatula anteriorly, holding it in his left hand, and carefully and gently he applies it laterally to the left infundibulopelvic ligament; he pushes the round ligament to the side. The infundibulopelvic ligament is now easily seen (Fig. 86).

The surgeon retrieves the abdominal end of the uterine tube with long tissue forceps and gently grasps both the ovary and the tube with an ovarian ring forceps. By pulling on the tube and ovary, he provides even better exposure of the infundibulopelvic ligament that is now tied off for the first time about 1–2 cm. above the abdominal extremity of the ovary. The suture is applied by means of a Deschamps aneurysm needle inserted from the medial side toward the lateral. To this end the operator draws the ovarian forceps sagittally so as to cause the infundibulopelvic ligament to be lifted somewhat from the pelvic wall, thereby reducing the potential danger to the underlying ureter (Fig. 87). While knotting this suture, however, the operator will find it appropriate to change the sagittal direction of the ovarian forceps to a horizontal one; this will be necessary because space is lacking for the manipulation required for knotting the catgut suture (Fig. 88). The surgeon can push the ligature upward easily with his index finger to cinch the knot. The end of the suture thread is left long and held in a clamp for later traction.

For security, one should religate the infundibulopelvic ligament a second time above the first suture (Fig. 89). This is accomplished by pulling down and left on both the ovarian ring forceps and the first ligature. The "safety ligature" is placed cephalad to the first; it is not left long, but cut short at once to ensure that no one will pull on it. If excessive traction should be exerted on the first ligature so that it comes off the stump, no harm is done because this safety ligature effectively prevents hemorrhage.

The doubly ligated infundibulopelvic ligament is now divided. The surgeon first repositions the ovarian forceps into a sagittal direction, causing the ligament to be lifted again away from the pelvic wall. The right assistant pulls the long end of the ligature upward with his left hand as the surgeon cuts across the ligament with scissors at a site between the ovary and the first suture just above the abdominal extremity of the ovary. Then the right assistant releases the round ligament being held with his anterolateral spatula. The retractor is repositioned laterally to the round ligament and the peritoneum is pushed to the side. The adnexa can now be easily mobilized caudally with a tug on the ovarian ring forceps, particularly since the infundibulopelvic ligament has already been severed, and the round ligament exposed (Fig. 90). The round ligament is sutured about 3–4 cm. above its junction with the uterus, the ligature being applied from the medial side by a Deschamps needle. The suture is left long for traction.

Blood vessels are sometimes encountered in the peritoneal reflection of the broad ligament between the round and the infun-

Figure 85.

Schauta-Amreich procedure. Anteverting the uterus. The bowel is packed back with a gauze strip. The right assistant lifts the bladder and loops of bowel with an intraperitoneal retractor. The peritoneal opening is stretched with two additional lateral spatulas. The uterine fundus is grasped with a double-toothed tenaculum and tilted forward out of the abdominal cavity. The adnexa are visible on the posterior surface of the inverted uterus.

See illustration on opposite page.

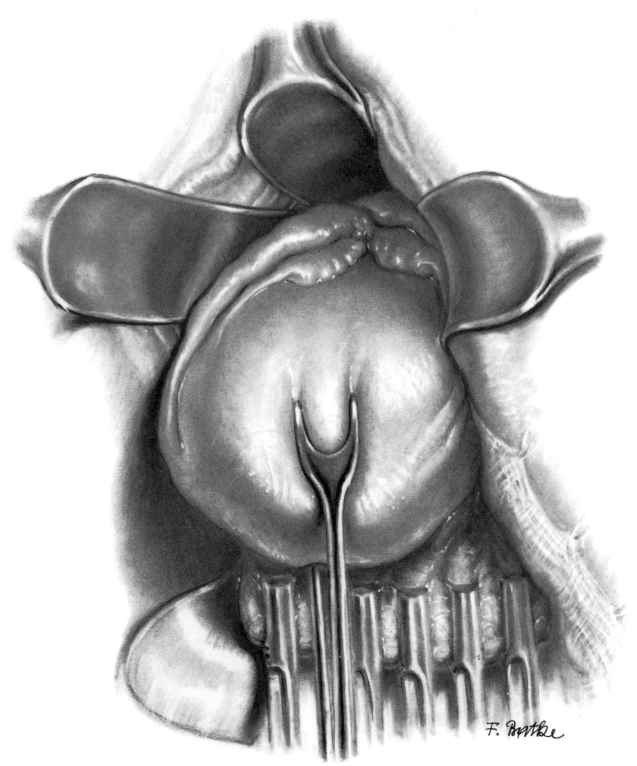

Figure 85. *See legend on opposite page.*

dibulopelvic ligaments. Therefore, before the ligated round ligament is divided, it should be resutured together with the infundibulopelvic ligament. This is done by pulling both ligaments down and to the left so that they can be jointly retied once again well above previously placed ligatures (Fig. 91). This second safety suture is also cut short and not used for traction. Now with the lower ligature pulled upward by the left assistant, the round ligament is cut across with scissors distally to the ligatures (Fig. 92). This effectively completes the division of the left adnexa from the pelvic wall, leaving relationships with the uterus intact.

Division of the Left Infundibulopelvic and Round Ligaments

First, the right-side assistant retracts bladder and bowel to the right and upward with the intraperitoneal spatula while pulling the

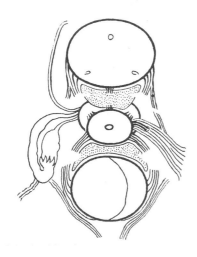

Figure 86.

Schauta-Amreich procedure. Preparing the field for dissection of the right adnexa. The left assistant pulls the anteverted uterine corpus down to the left by means of the claw tenaculum, turning it somewhat clockwise. In addition, he pushes the bladder and the packed bowel up to the left with an anterior spatula. The right assistant retracts the round ligament laterally with a spatula in his left hand. Thus, the right adnexa have been appropriately prepared for dissection as diagrammed above.

See illustration on opposite page.

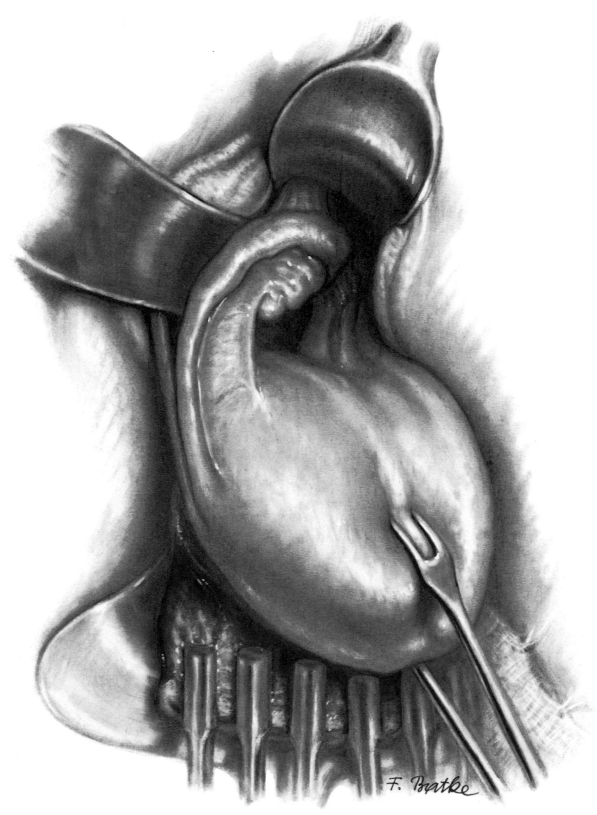

Figure 86. *See legend on opposite page.*

uterus and the vaginal cuff to the right and downward. The round ligament is pushed laterally by the left assistant with a lateral retractor that he holds in his right hand. The operator grasps the tube and the ovary with a ring forceps, positioning it sagittally; then he ligates the infundibulopelvic ligament that has been lifted away from the pelvic sidewall. It is sutured with a Deschamps ligature carrier passed through from the medial side.

Once again, in order to gain space for use while tying the knot, the ovarian ring forceps is laid flat against the pelvic wall by the right assistant, using his right hand. To ensure that blood loss will be minimal, a second ligature is now placed on the infundibulopelvic ligament proximally to the first. Then the ligament is divided distally to both sutures. Next the round ligament is released from the right lateral spatula and is ligated with the suture applied from the lateral side. Both the infundibulopelvic and the round ligaments are now jointly religated, and the round ligament is severed.

Figure 87.

Schauta-Amreich procedure. First ligation of the infundibulopelvic ligament (ligamentum suspensorium ovarii). The tubes and ovaries have been grasped with ovum forceps and are pulled downward to the left by the surgeon's left hand. The right assistant pushes the round ligament far to the side with a spatula to expose the infundibulopelvic ligament medially. The infundibulopelvic ligament is ligated now for the first time using a Deschamps aneurysm needle inserted from the medial side. Note that the ovarian ring forceps lifts the adnexa somewhat away from the pelvic wall, reducing the risk of damaging the ureter, which is located here, during the infundibulopelvic ligation.

See illustration on opposite page.

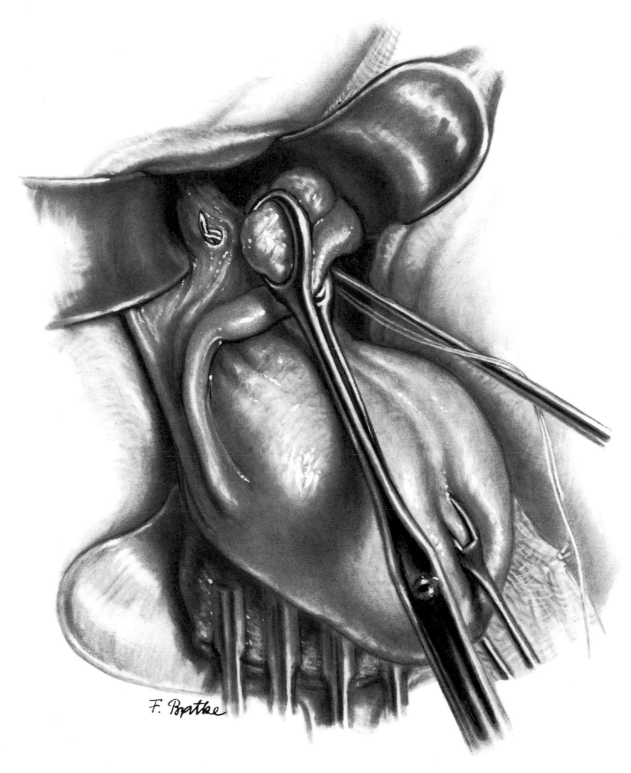

Figure 87. *See legend on opposite page.*

The long ends of the sutures on the stumps of the infundibulo-pelvic and the round ligaments are laid on the abdomen together. The uterus is attached now only by the lateral parametria.

These two ligaments can also be divided between clamps. However, one should be advised against this practice because (1) the clamps can come off the severed ligaments or even tear off before they are securely sutured; (2) should it become necessary to clamp the ligaments high up, the closely underlying ureter may be injured by the clamp (a situation unlikely to occur when ligating with a Deschamps carrier under direct vision); and (3) the ligaments have to be severed after clamping even before a "safety ligature" can be applied.

Figure 88.

Schauta-Amreich procedure. Ligating the infundibulopelvic ligament. The left assistant retracts the bowel with an intraperitoneal spatula and pulls the corpus uteri down to the left with the tenaculum. The right assistant pushes the round ligament aside to prepare the right infundibulopelvic ligament for ligation. When the ligature is being tied, the ring forceps are held horizontally by the right assistant's right hand and applied against the posterior uterine wall. Thus, the surgeon increases the space available for tying the ligature high up in the operative field without difficulty.

See illustration on opposite page.

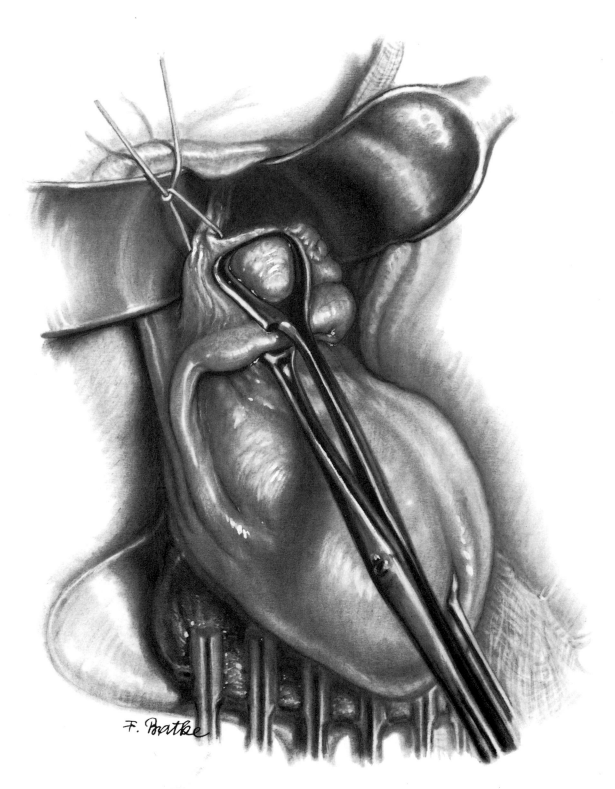

Figure 88. *See legend on opposite page.*

Technical Problems

1. If too much tissue is incorporated into the Deschamps suture while ligating the infundibulopelvic ligament, the ureter lying nearby beneath the peritoneal-covered ligaments can also be ligated.

2. The first ligature on the infundibulopelvic ligament may be placed too closely to the abdominal extremity of the ovary so that the ligature is too near the cut edge of the stump when it is divided. If this occurs, the suture may come off the ligamentous stump at the least pull.

Figure 89.

Schauta-Amreich procedure. Religation of the infundibulopelvic ligament. The operative field is prepared and the right round ligament is pushed aside. The right infundibulopelvic ligament has been ligated and the suture ends left long; it is retracted down to the left by the surgeon, who pulls with regulated force on the ring forceps. The infundibulopelvic ligament is ligated again above the first ligature with the Deschamps needle applied from the medial side. It should be emphasized that the ring forceps attached to the right adnexa are again placed sagittally and lifted from the pelvic wall to avoid ligating the ureter while ligating the infundibulopelvic ligament.

See illustration on opposite page.

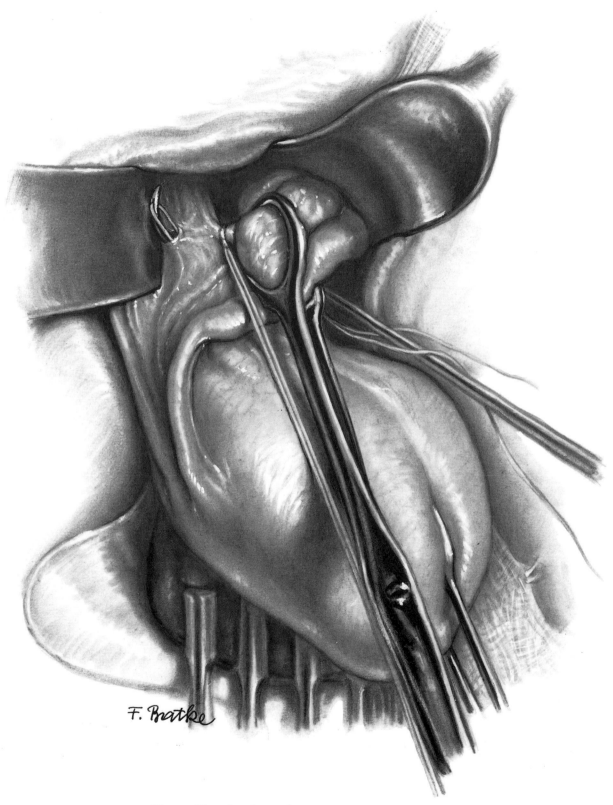

Figure 89.   *See legend on opposite page.*

3. It may not be possible to place a second tie on the infundibulopelvic ligament by virtue of technical difficulties. A second safety ligature is always to be preferred even if it has to be affixed closely above the first one. If only one is placed, however, and it comes off either because of a strong pull or poor purchase, massive hemorrhage will occur from the ovarian artery and vein. These vessels retract into the infundibulopelvic ligament and it is then very difficult, if not impossible, to grasp them again with a clamp. There is additional hazard because of the proximity of the ureter to the cranial portion of the ligament. In order to staunch bleeding from these retracted vessels in the infundibulopelvic ligament, laparotomy may be necessary. However, in a series of over 800 Schauta-Amreich radical procedures done to date, this complication was never encountered because it was always possible to place the second infundibulopelvic ligature.

Figure 90.

Schauta-Amreich procedure. Ligating the round ligament (ligamentum teres uteri). The infundibulopelvic ligament is doubly ligated and divided. The cephalad ligature is cut short and the long end of the caudal suture is held upward. The right assistant takes the ring forceps from the surgeon and holds it down to the left with his right hand; additionally, he releases the round ligament, retracting the peritoneum located laterally to the round ligament with the spatula instead. A ligature is placed about the round ligament from the medial side with a Deschamps needle.

See illustration on opposite page.

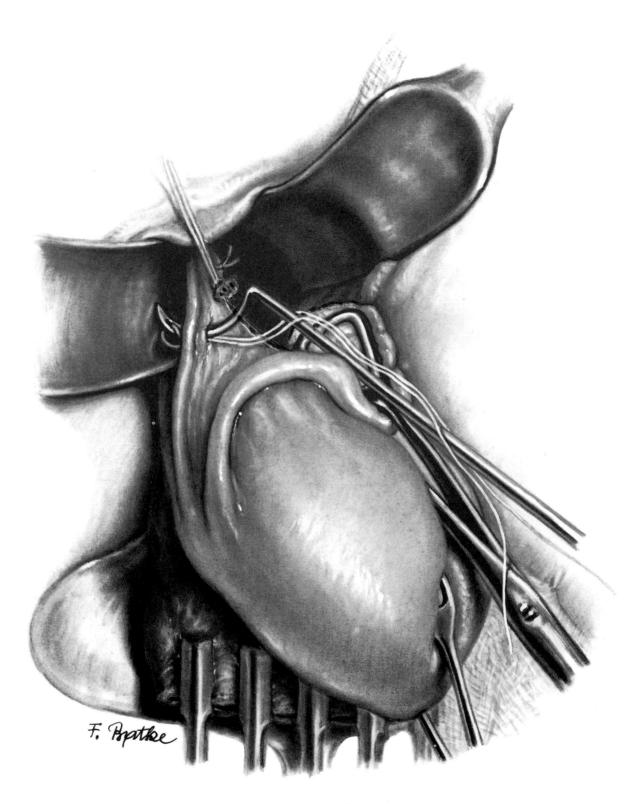

F. Pspatke

Figure 90.   *See legend on opposite page.*

Technique

For purposes of resecting the right parametrium, the operative field is prepared as follows (Fig. 93): The left assistant vigorously advances bladder and loops of bowel up to the left with a right-angled retractor inserted anteriorly into the peritoneal cavity, while also pulling the vaginal cuff and the uterine fundus by the attached clamps to the left. The right-side assistant pushes the ureter upward with a long, narrow spatula in the right paravesical space and with a broader, shorter spatula in the right pararectal space, he retracts the vaginal wall strongly to the right.

The surgeon visually checks to ensure that the right ureter is well up out of the way and is protected by the spatula. Inserting a long, narrow spatula into the culdesac of Douglas, he depresses the forward-ballooning rectum toward the sacrum. The right parametrium is now clearly exposed as a wide tissue layer coursing diagonally from the edge of the cervix upward and out to the pelvic wall (Fig. 93). One or more curved parametrial clamps can be placed at the lateral base of the parametrium close to the sidewall. Then the tissue is divided with scissors in stepwise fashion from its caudal edge cranially.

All the steps are repeated analogously on the left side: the right assistant pulls the uterus and the vaginal cuff down to the right and pushes the bowel and bladder up and right with the right-angled retractor. The left assistant holds back the ureter toward the left paravesical space and pushes the vaginal wall laterally toward the pararectal space. The surgeon depresses the rectum and dissects the left Mackinrodt ligament by the clamp method close to the pelvic wall. The cardinal ligament can also be separated from the pelvic wall with no prior clamping, yet without incurring substantial bleeding. This is the case because both the uterine and the middle hemorrhoidal arteries have previously been ligated. Anomalous vessels, often encountered in the areas supplied by the peripheral branches of the pelvic vessels, can result in diffuse bleeding, especially venous in origin. Therefore, clamping the cardinal ligament before dividing it is preferable to free dissection.

Technical Problems

1. Insufficient mobilization or inadequate displacement of the ureter may cause the ureter to be caught in the tip of the uppermost parametrial clamp. Before the parametrial clamp is closed and before the lateral parametrium is divided, it is absolutely necessary to recheck the ureteral course visually again.

2. The parametrial clamps must not be seated too high up on the pelvic wall or else one can injure large blood vessels in this area.

3. The anteriorly-ballooning rectum has to be pushed down toward the sacrum with a long retractor. If not, it can get in the way of the scissors during the lateral parametrial dissection.

SUTURING THE PARAMETRIUM

The parametrial clamps are replaced by catgut suture-ligatures. In ligating the parametrium close to the large pelvic-wall vessels, one must proceed with special care so as to avoid injuring the thin-walled veins. Tissues in the most distal clamp are ligated first; the needle is gently inserted close to the tip of the clamp. While the ligature is being knotted, the assistant should open the clamp slowly as the surgeon simultaneously cinches the suture with even pressure. A triple surgical knot is recommended.

As the uppermost parametrial clamp is being replaced, the site at which the needle is inserted at the tip of the clamp must be kept in constant view to ascertain with absolute certainty that the ureter is well out of the way. Even though the ureter may not be directly punctured during ligation, it can still be pulled up and tented as the suture is tied if it has not been displaced enough. If this occurs, the ureter must then be pushed somewhat upward from the ligature with the closed scissors.

CLOSURE OF THE PERITONEAL CAVITY

Placing the Pseudo-angle Suture

The anterior edge of the peritoneum is pushed upward to the right, together with the bowel, by means of an intraperitoneal right-angled retractor held by the right assistant, who is simultaneously pulling the suture attached to the posterior peritoneal edge down to the right. The left assistant pulls the stay-sutures on the stumps of the left infundibulopelvic and round ligaments upward with his right hand, while retracting the left ureter up with a longer lateral spatula held in his left hand. The surgeon identifies the edge of the peritoneal slit at the lateral pelvic wall approximately at the level of the uterine vascular stump; this represents the uppermost pseudo-angle of the peritoneal opening at the medial base of the rectal pillar (Fig. 94). A catgut suture is inserted here (Fig. 95); its ends are left long and held in a clamp for traction. The ureteral knee is pushed slightly away from this angle suture with the closed scissors (Fig. 96).

Inserting the Peritoneal Angle Suture

The angle of the peritoneal wound is now sutured on the left while the stumps are simultaneously extraperitonealized. To accomplish this a half purse-string suture is carried out beginning anteriorly at the left side. The right assistant vigorously pushes the bowel and the anterior peritoneal wound edge upward to the right of the symphysis with a wide intraperitoneal retractor in his left hand; this he does by turning the right-angle retractor strongly counterclockwise so that the surface of the retractor blade is almost in a sagittal plane, thereby stretching the left half of the anterior peritoneal wound edge. With his right hand he pulls the posterior peritoneal traction suture down to the right. The left assistant depresses the sutures attached to the stumps of the round and infundibulopelvic ligaments and those on the pseudo-angle to the left with his left hand; he also lifts the ureter to the left in the left paravesical space with a lateral spatula in his right hand.

(Text continued on page 190)

Figure 94.

Schauta-Amreich procedure. Preparing the left peritoneal angle for closing the peritoneum. The right assistant holds back the bowel with a long gauze pack which he retracts upward and to the right with a wide right-angled spatula, pulling the silk traction suture attached to the posterior peritoneal wound edge downward. The left assistant elevates the freed ureter with a long lateral spatula and pulls the traction suture on the infundibulopelvic and round ligaments upward with his right hand. The uterus is removed together with the adnexa and the parametrium. The left peritoneal angle is exposed. One can recognize the ureteral knee, the ligated uterine vascular pedicle medially to it and the stumps of the infundibulopelvic and round ligaments pulled upward. Laterally to the ureteral knee at the pelvic wall is seen the ligated parametrial stump; caudally is the ligated stump of the rectal pillar adherent to the rectal peritoneum.

See illustration on opposite page.

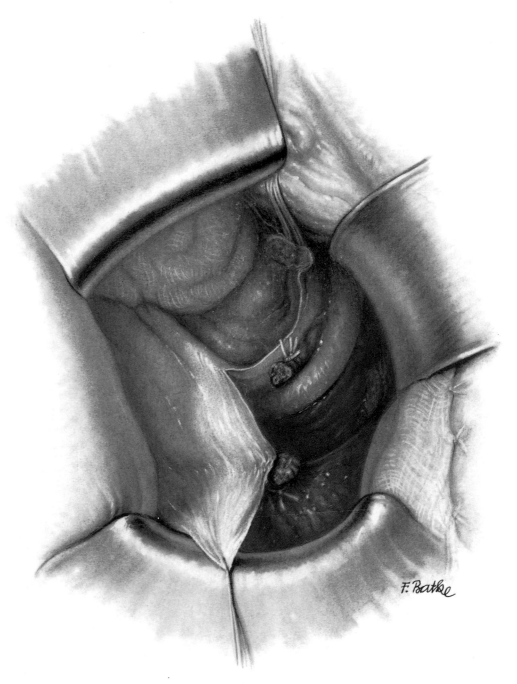

Figure 94.   *See legend on opposite page.*

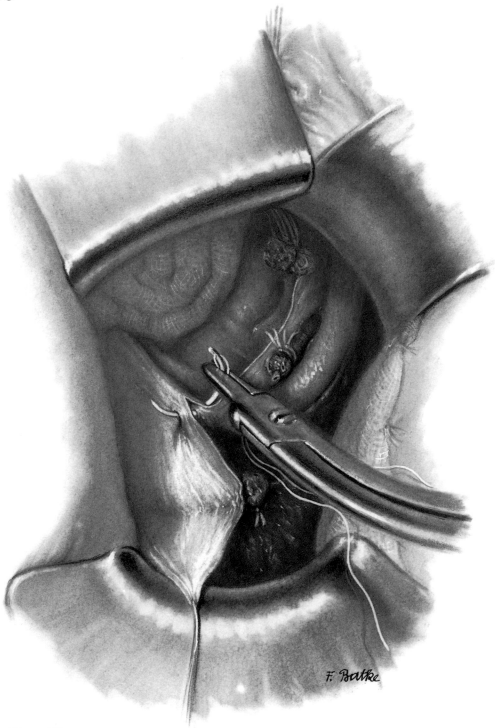

Figure 95.

Schauta-Amreich procedure. Placing the left peritoneal pseudo-angle suture. The operative field is prepared as in Figure 94. Medially to the ureteral knee, a triangular incision is found at the peritoneal wound edge; it is closed by a single suture. The surgeon grasps the uppermost peritoneal wound angle in the needle.

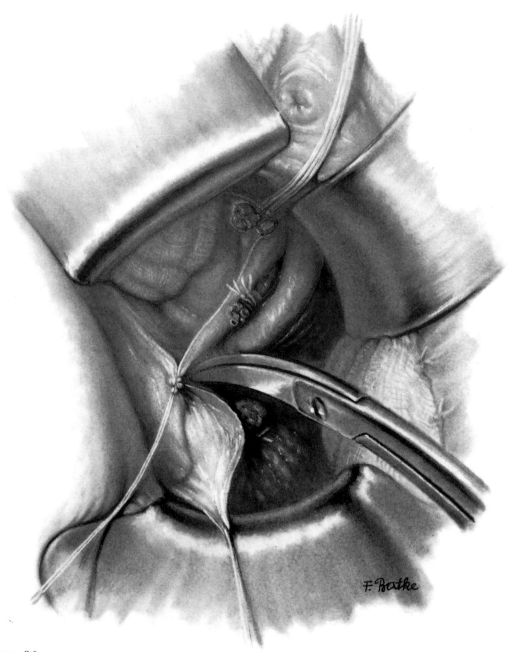

Figure 96.

Schauta-Amreich procedure. Displacing the ureteral knee during peritoneal closure. The pseudo-angle suture on the left side is tied. The closely adherent ureteral knee is pushed upward with the closed scissors, thus mobilizing it once again.

The surgeon can now identify the left uppermost angle of the peritoneal wound edge. A purse-string suture is placed from above down as follows: First, he inserts the needle through the anterior peritoneal edge starting from the outside; then he passes it through the peritoneum overlying the infundibulopelvic and round ligament stumps; next, the uppermost corner of the peritoneal wound angle is grasped (Fig. 97). At this point, the left assistant changes the direction of pull on the infundibulopelvic and round ligaments as well as on the pseudo-angle suture, drawing them upward and left. With the lateral spatula in his left hand he pushes the lateral vaginal wall extraperitoneally to the side. (The left assistant changes hands, substituting the stay-sutures for the spatula, at first pulling the suture ends down with his left hand and elevating the ureter with the spatula in his right hand, and then later drawing the sutures up with his right hand and retracting the vaginal wall laterally with the spatula in his left hand). Now the left peritoneal edge is exposed so that the suturing may continue medially to the uterine vascular stump, moving somewhat caudad to it, and finally grasping the peritoneum at the rectum (Fig. 98).

(Text continued on page 194)

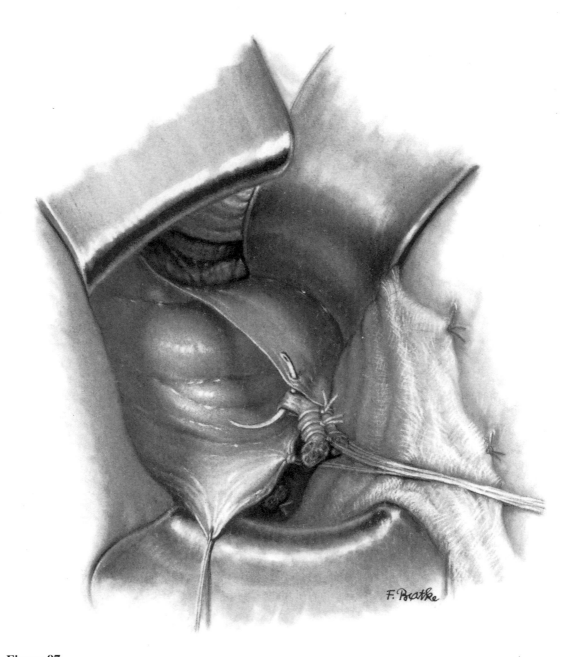

Figure 97.

   Schauta-Amreich procedure. Placement of the left angle suture for closing the peritoneum. The right assistant pushes the bowel up to the right with the large intraperitoneal right-angled retractor. The left assistant pulls the traction sutures on the round and infundibulopelvic ligaments to the left along with the suture on the pseudo-angle; he also elevates the bladder with an anterolateral spatula applied extraperitoneally. The surgeon initiates the left peritoneal angle suture by first placing the needle through the anterior peritoneal cut edge and then through the peritoneum over the infundibulopelvic stump, sewing from above down.

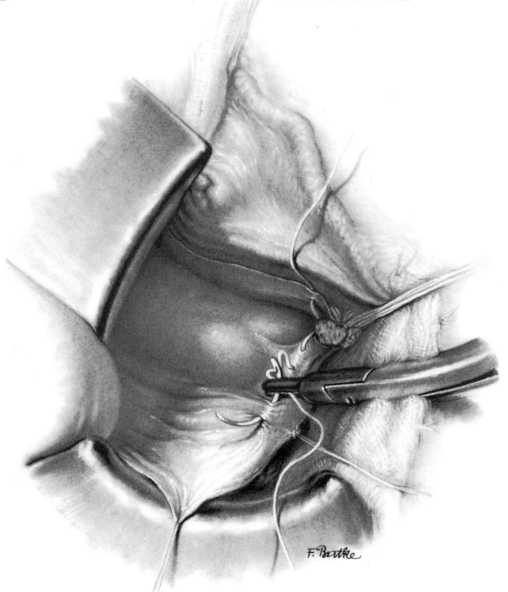

Figure 98.

Schauta-Amreich procedure. Continuing the left peritoneal angle suture. The bowel is retracted upward by the right-side assistant using a wide intraperitoneal spatula; at the same time he pulls down on the traction suture attached to the posterior peritoneal edge. The left assistant pulls the sutures on the round and infundibulopelvic stumps up and left, while pulling down and left on the pseudo-angle suture. The peritoneal angle suture, begun anteriorly, is continued around to include the peritoneum medially to the ureter and over the rectum; the needle should come out near the pseudo-angle suture. If high peritonealization is desired, the suture must be placed at the posterior peritoneal edge.

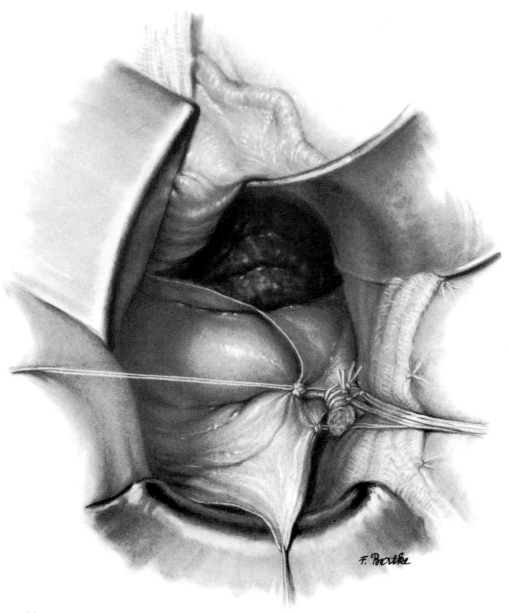

Figure 99.

    Schauta-Amreich procedure. Tying the left angle suture. The left assistant pushes the bladder up with an anterolateral spatula and draws aside the sutures attached to the infundibulopelvic and round ligaments and the pseudo-angle. The left angle suture is tied; it lies somewhat cephalad and medially to the pseudo-angle suture (in high peritonealization as shown). The stumps are thereby extraperitonealized. The angle suture has been pulled medially for exposure.

This concludes the left half of the purse-string suture that can now be tied. This is done with the left assistant pulling the round and infundibulopelvic stumps laterally while the right assistant relaxes his grasp a little on the posterior peritoneal edge and loosens his grip on the anterior intraperitoneal retractor so that the peritoneum is no longer under tension. The surgeon ties the half purse-string suture at this time, and thereby he closes the entire left side of the peritoneal opening (Fig. 99). The long end of the pseudo-angle suture is cut, leaving the left assistant holding only the newly-placed left angle suture.

Next, the surgeon executes another peritoneal suture to bring together the anterior edge, sewing from the outside in, and the posterior edge, from the inside out. This apposes both peritoneal cut edges on the left side a second time. The long end of the left corner suture can now be cut short.

If a rectocele coexists, then high peritonealization will be needed. Accordingly, the anterior peritoneal wound edge is not brought together with the posterior edge, but the peritoneum in the culdesac of Douglas is taken considerably higher up instead.

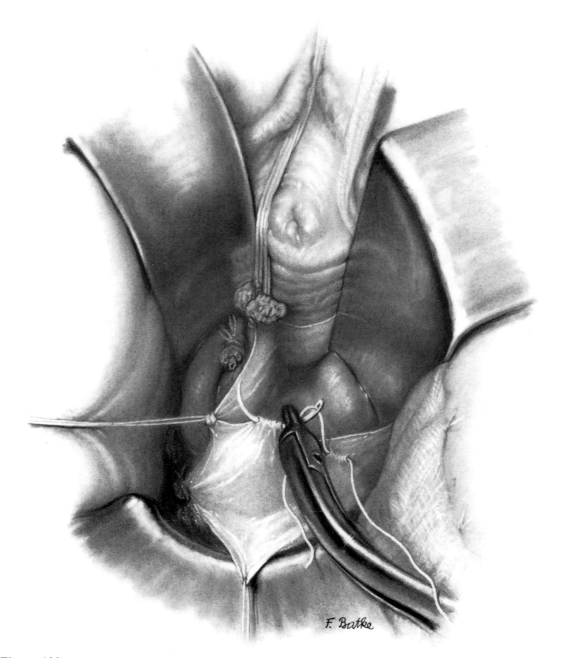

Figure 100.

Schauta-Amreich procedure. Placing the right peritoneal angle suture. The left-side assistant lifts the bowel to the left with a large right-angled retractor and pulls the posterior peritoneal edge down by its attached silk suture. The right assistant pulls the right pseudo-angle suture to the side, elevating the ureter upward with an anterolateral spatula extraperitoneally. The traction sutures on the infundibulopelvic and round ligaments are placed on the patient's abdomen. Medially to the ureter, one can see the uterine vascular pedicle; caudad to the ureteral knee at the lateral edge of the peritoneum is the stump of the rectal pillar. The surgeon begins the right peritoneal angle suture at the rectal peritoneum, picking it up on the needle somewhat medially to the pseudo-angle suture.

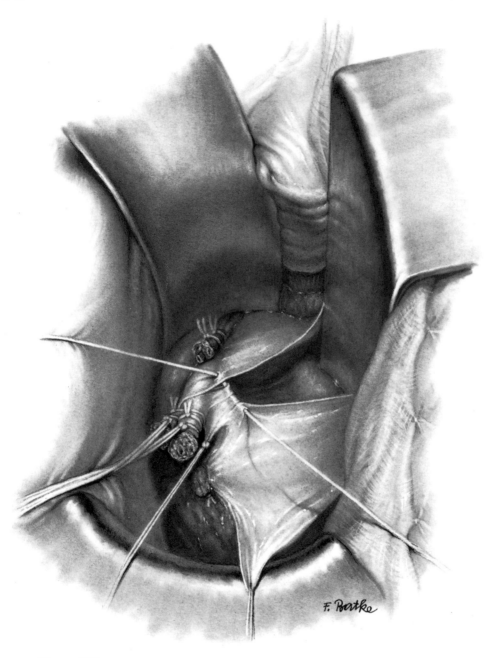

Figure 102.

    Schauta-Amreich procedure. Tying the right peritoneal angle suture. The operative field is prepared as in Figure 101. The right peritoneal angle suture is placed by sewing the edge from the rectum around to the anterior peritoneum. Note the high peritonealization that begins above the pseudo-angle suture and is continued medially to the infundibulopelvic ligament up to the anterior peritoneal edge, extraperitonealizing the stumps.

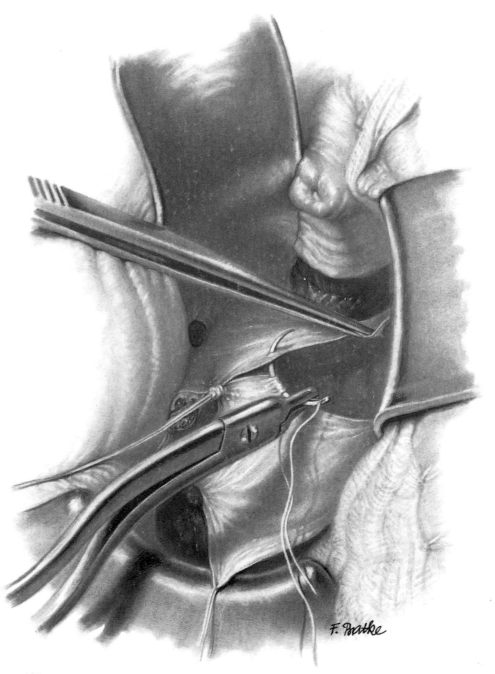

Figure 103.

Schauta-Amreich procedure. Continuing the peritoneal suture. The right peritoneal suture is tied and pulled downward to the right by the right assistant; he also pushes the bladder back extraperitoneally with an anterolateral spatula. The high peritonealization is continued medially to the right angle suture to unite the rectal peritoneum with the anterior peritoneal wound edge.

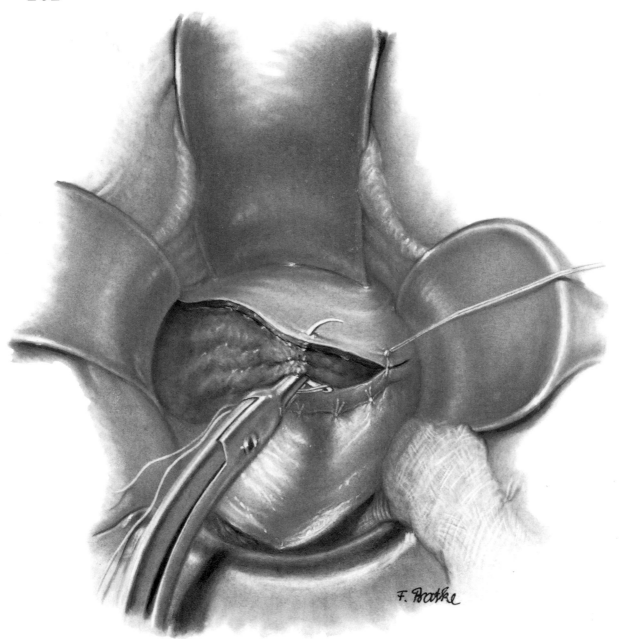

Figure 105.

Schauta-Amreich procedure. Plicating the bladder. The wound cavity is prepared with one anterior and two lateral spatulas as well as a self-retaining posterior retractor. The peritoneal cavity is closed. The transverse row of peritoneal sutures is visible on the left; they are covered by the descending bladder on the right. At the left side, the first bladder-plication suture has already been tied and pulled laterally by the left assistant. The operator places another plication suture at several sites in the bladder wall, fixing it to the anterior vaginal wound edge. This lifts the descended bladder.

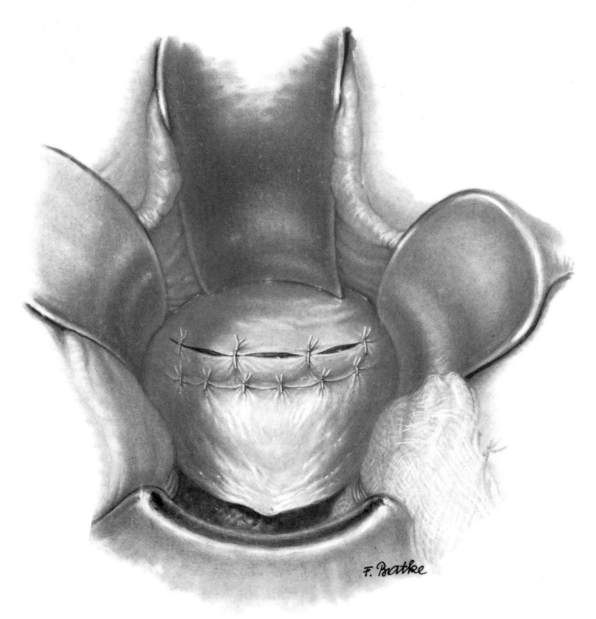

Figure 106.

Schauta-Amreich procedure. Appearance of the field at the peritoneal closing. The wound is exposed with four retractors. Two transverse rows of sutures are seen: the lower one corresponds to the peritoneal closing sutures; the upper, the bladder plication.

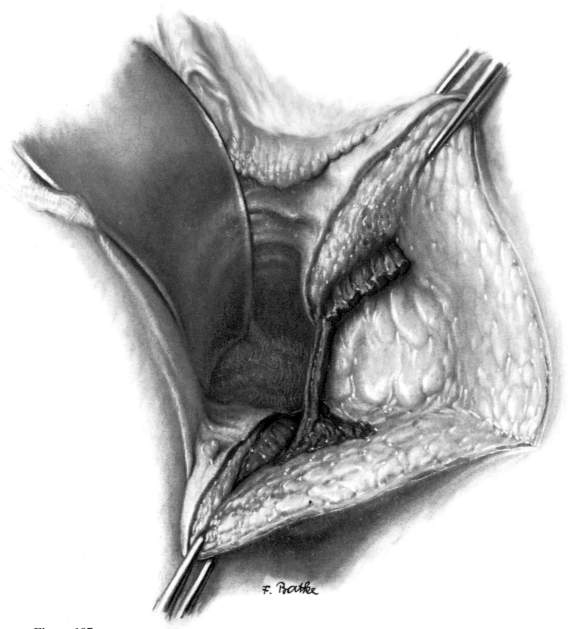

F. Batke

Figure 107.

Schauta-Amreich procedure. Preparing the wound site for closing the Schuchardt incision. The subperitoneal space is loosely tamponaded with a gauze pad. The right-side assistant spreads the vaginal canal with a spatula. The Schuchardt incision is stretched with two single-toothed tenacula placed on either side of the posterior commissure. Deep down in the gaping wound one sees the partially severed levator muscle.

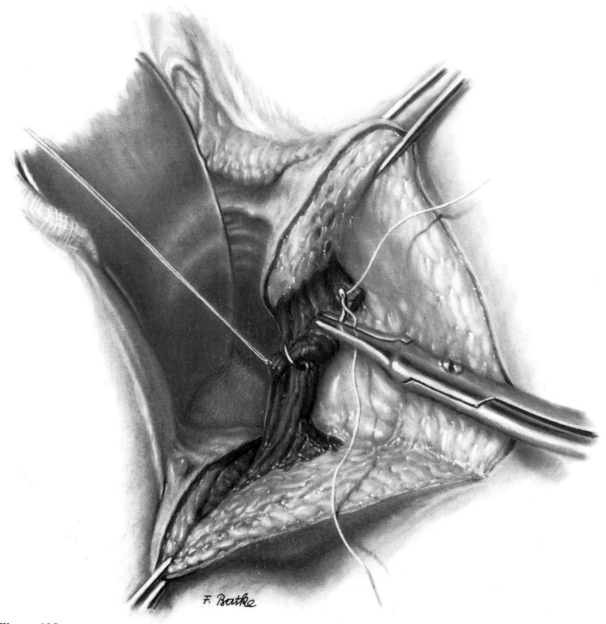

Figure 108.

Schauta-Amreich procedure. Uniting the levator muscle. The uppermost levator suture has already been tied. The levator wound edges are united by another suture.

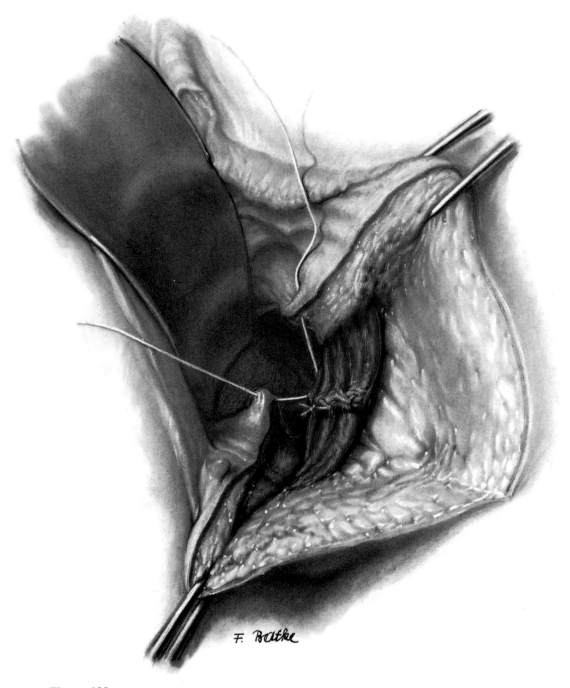

Figure 109.

Schauta-Amreich procedure. Apposing the vaginal wound edge. The levator muscle is sewn. In uniting the vaginal mucosal edges, one begins at the uppermost angle of the wound where the longitudinal incision meets the circumferential incision. It is important to include the levator muscle in the depth of the topmost suture of the vaginal edges in order to prevent subperitoneal serous secretions from flowing down from above to reach the Schuchardt wound.

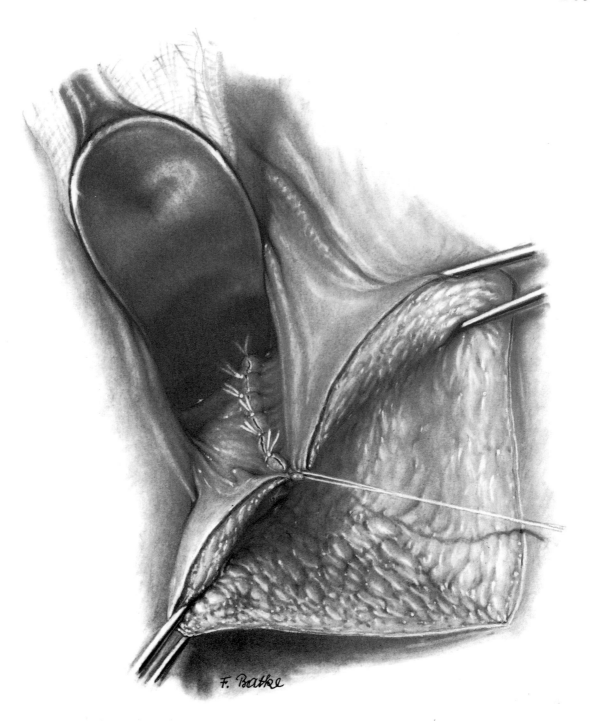

Figure 110.

Schauta-Amreich procedure. Suturing the vaginal wound. The longitudinal incision of the vagina is sutured down to the posterior commissure with catgut. The ends of the last suture are left long for traction.

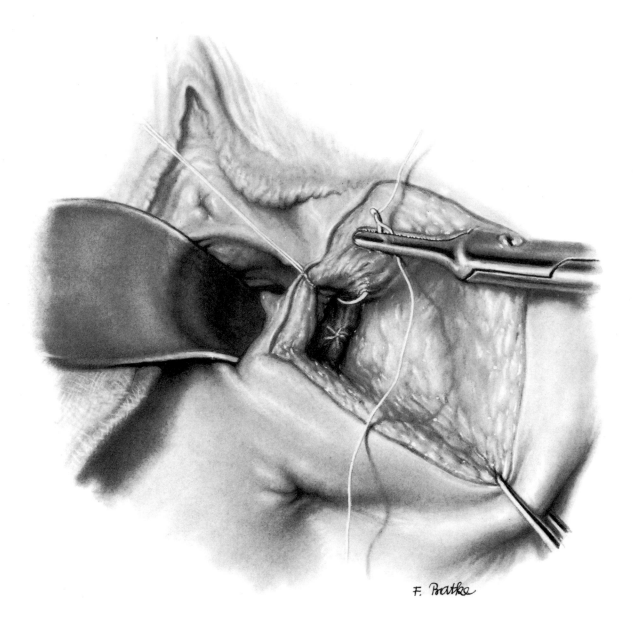

Figure 111.

Schauta-Amreich procedure. Sewing the bulbocavernosus muscle. The right assistant spreads the vagina with a retractor and pulls the last vaginal suture upward and to the right. The tenacula on the posterior commissure are removed. One single-toothed tenaculum is placed at the lowest angle of the perineal skin and is pulled downward to the left by the left assistant. The surgeon sutures the bulbocavernosus muscle over the united levator muscle seen deep down in the wound.

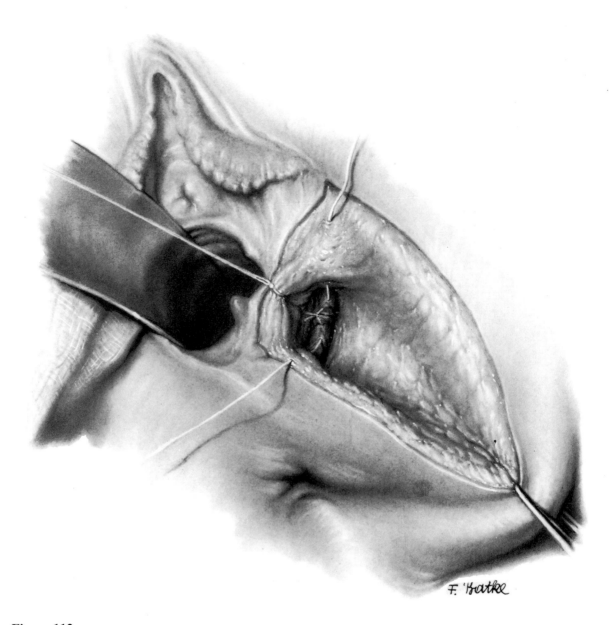

Figure 112.

Schauta-Amreich procedure. Suturing the bulbocavernosus muscle and the urogenital diaphragm. In order to avoid forming dead space while reconstructing the pelvic floor, the levator muscle (at the depths) and the fibers of the urogenital diaphragm (medially) should be incorporated into the bulbocavernosus suture.

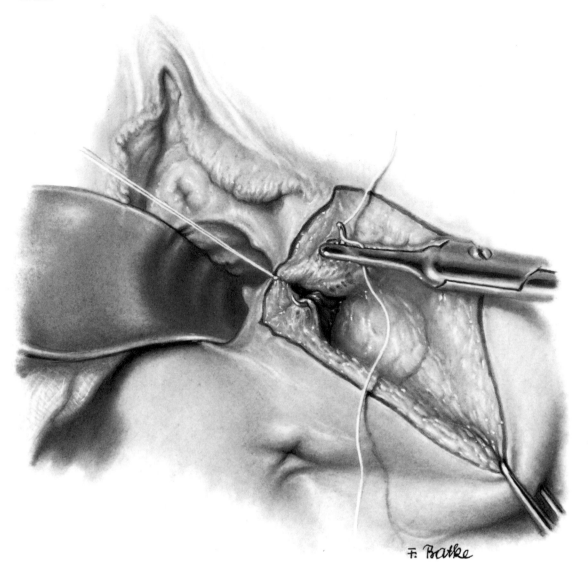

Figure 113.

   Schauta-Amreich procedure. Closing the perineum in layers. Several rows of sutures are placed and tied to join the deep tissues of the perineum.

Figure 114.

   Schauta-Amreich procedure. Coapting the skin edges. The perineal skin edges are joined with interrupted silk sutures. At the posterior commissure can be seen the last vaginal suture that was placed. An indwelling catheter is inserted into the bladder (and the balloon inflated). The upper vaginal wound has been loosely tamponaded with a gauze packing.

See illustration on opposite page

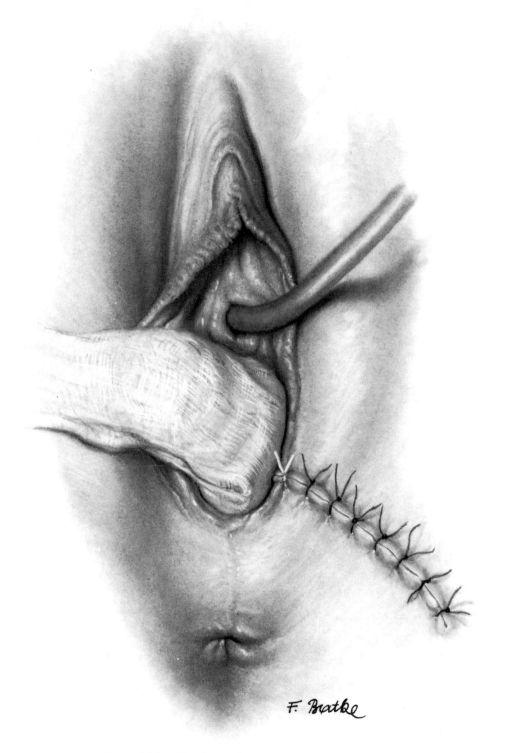

Figure 114. *See legend on opposite page.*

VAGINAL HYSTERECTOMY

CIRCUMCISION OF THE VAGINAL CANAL

The vaginal circumcision provides access to the vesicovaginal and the rectovaginal spaces. After these two spaces have been opened, additional dissection will displace the bladder and the rectum. Then the plica vesicouterina and the culdesac of Douglas can be opened to allow separation of the para-tissues from the uterus.

Technique

The vagina is exposed with four retractors: the anterior and the right spatulas are held by the right assistant; the posterior and the left, by the left assistant. The surgeon places two single-toothed tenacula on the anterior lip of the cervix and another on the posterior lip. He pulls the uterus down by means of these tenacula. The anterior circumcision is carried out in the anterior fornix at a site immediately above the transition of the smooth wall of the portio vaginalis of the cervix into the wrinkled vaginal wall mucosa. This border is identified by moving the tenacula on the portio up and down.

The circumcision is begun in the anterior inverted vaginal wall in a bow-shaped incision, elongated bilaterally where it curves somewhat upward (Fig. 115). The depth of the incision reaches at first only through the vaginal mucosa; it is properly executed when the wound gapes merely as a result of the pressure being applied by

---

Figure 115.

Vaginal hysterectomy. Anterior vaginal circumcision. The vagina is spread by one anterior, two lateral and one self-retaining posterior retractors. The anterior and right spatulas are held by the right assistant and the left by the left assistant. The anterior lip of the cervix is grasped with two single-toothed tenacula, the posterior lip with one tenaculum. The surgeon pulls the uterus down by means of these tenacula. The anterior circumcision is begun in the vaginal fornix and reaches higher laterally. With proper upward pressure on the anterior spatula and incision in the correct depth, the vaginal wound gapes.

214

See illustration on opposite page.

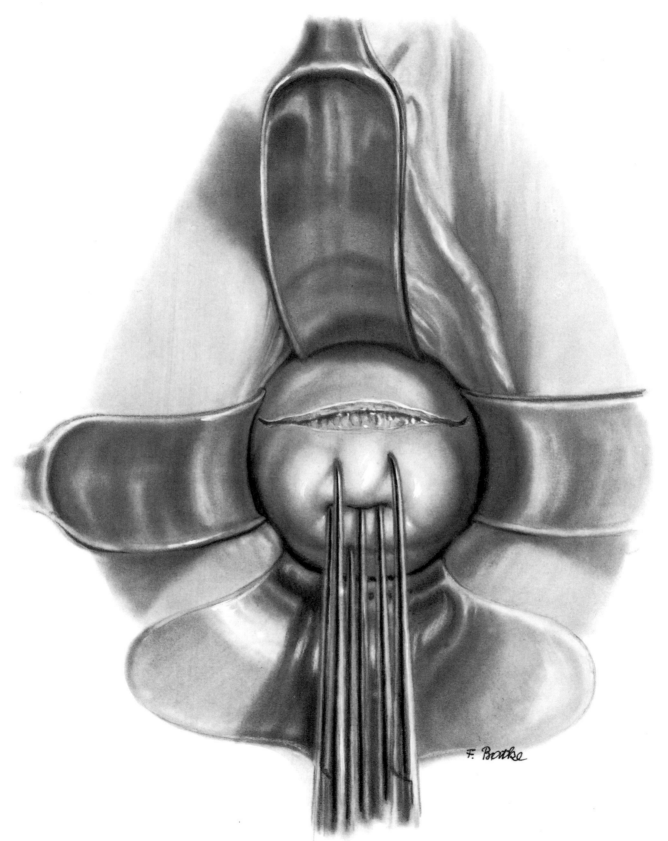

Figure 115. *See legend on opposite page.*

the anterior spatula. Subsequently, the anterior midline tissues are severed to penetrate the fascia vaginalis and open the vesicovaginal space.

By appropriate upward spatula pressure, the bladder and its covering fascia are elevated until the fibers of the supravaginal septum are stretched. In the most lateral aspects of the circumcision, only the mucosa is cut, leaving the fascia vaginalis intact and undamaged here. To carry out the incision laterally through the fascia vaginalis, might open the vaginal outflow veins located in the fascia, causing severe hemorrhage.

The surgeon then passes the tenacula, which are attached to the portio, to the right assistant. He in turn holds them in his left hand and stretches the inverted vaginal wall by pulling the uterus upward. The posterior circumcision of the vaginal canal is executed through the posterior fornix. It begins at the right end of the anterior incision and courses in a bow shape across the posterior fornix to meet the left end of the anterior incision (Fig. 116). This circumcises the vagina.

Both the mucosa and the vaginal fascia are cut in the midline posteriorly, but laterally only the mucosa is incised. The lateral parts of the circumcision serve only to demarcate where the parametrial sutures will be anchored later. Medially in the posterior circumcision, the fascia must be severed in order for the rectovaginal space and the culdesac of Douglas to be prepared and opened.

Technical Problems

1. If the incision is made too far anteriorly in the portio rather than in the vaginal fornix, one cannot open the vesicovaginal space nor can the supravaginal space be reached. Moreover, the lower bladder pole will be fixed to the anterior cervix in the vesicovaginal space by dense connective tissue, making it difficult to separate the bladder from the cervix later.

2. When the circumcision is done too superficially so that the vaginal fascia is not penetrated, the vesicovaginal space is not entered. As a result attempts to dissect the lower bladder pole may result in damage to the bladder by virtue of the fact that one is dissecting too close to it.

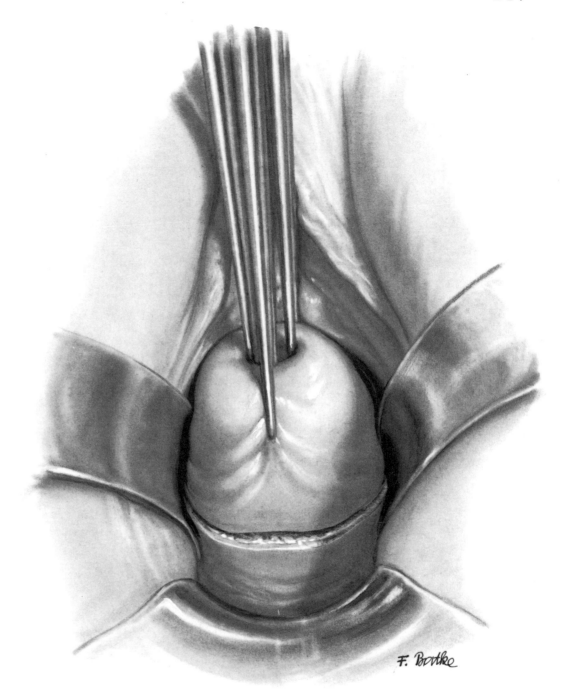

Figure 116.

Vaginal hysterectomy. Posterior vaginal circumcision. The field is prepared with one posterior and two lateral spatulas; the right assistant pulls the uterus upward by means of the tenaculum in his left hand. With counterpressure on the posterior self-retaining retractor, the inverted posterior vaginal wall is placed on stretch and can be incised circularly in the posterior fornix, joining the anterior circumcisional wound at the sides.

3. If the circumcision is carried too deeply in the lateral aspects so that the vaginal fascia is penetrated, bleeding will ensue from injuries to the veins of the vaginal plexus coursing in the lateral vaginal fascia.

4. Circumcision done too near the portio in the posterior fornix places the operator close to the cervix and in the wrong tissue layer, so that the culdesac of Douglas is found only with great difficulty. He may think the problem is due to adhesions, but this is not the case; instead, he has been deluded by the original error in dissection.

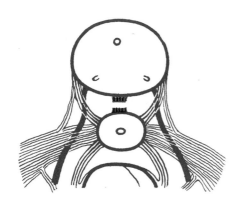

Figure 117.

Vaginal hysterectomy. Division of the supravaginal septum. The incision in the anterior vaginal wall is carried through the fascia vaginalis in the midline to enter the vesicocervical space. The tenacula on the anterior lip of the cervix are repositioned so that they grasp the anterior vaginal wound edge and make the wound gape more. The left assistant pulls the uterus down firmly via the tenacula; both assistants retract the vaginal walls laterally with the spatulas. The bladder is elevated with upward pressure on the anterior spatula by the right assistant. Thus, the fibers of the supravaginal fascia, which course from the anterior surface of the cervix to the lower pole of the bladder, are stretched. The surgeon lifts up the lower pole of the bladder with toothed tissue forceps and dissects these tensely stretched fibers of the supravaginal septum near the cervix. The tips of the curved dissecting scissors should point toward the cervix. This step is shown schematically above.

See illustration on opposite page.

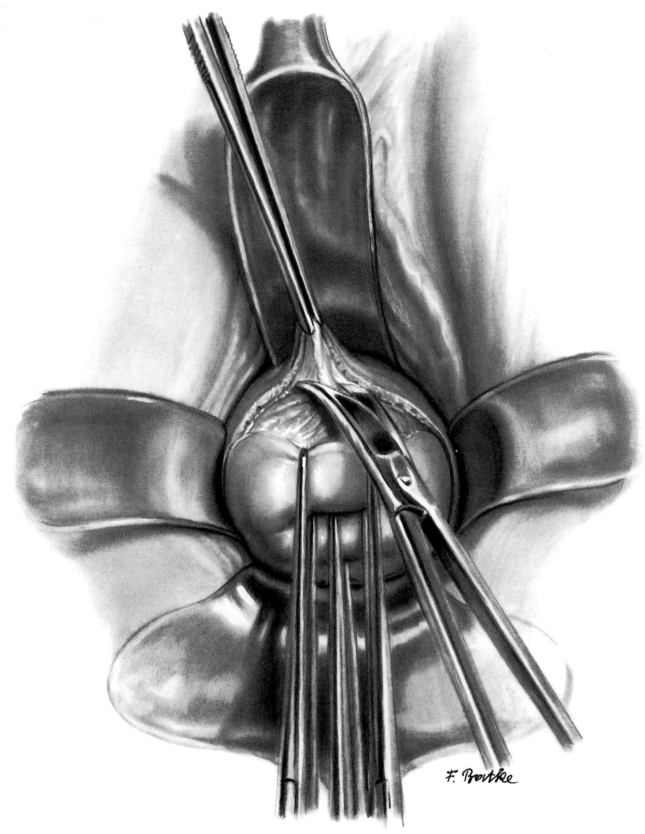

Figure 117. *See legend on opposite page.*

DISSECTION OF THE URINARY BLADDER

Technique

Tenacula are placed on the portio to grasp the anterior lip radially across from within the cervical canal to the anterior vaginal circumcision wound edge, thus causing the vaginal wound to gape still more (Fig. 117). By pulling the tenacula down in combination with appropriate upward pressure on the anterior spatula, one can stretch the fibers of the supravaginal septum (these fibers fix the lower pole of the bladder to the anterior wall of the cervix). Such fibers must always be sharply dissected and this is best done with one or more scissor cuts. To accomplish this the surgeon picks up the lower bladder pole with tissue forceps and pulls it up and somewhat toward himself, cutting the stretched fibers just caudad to the forceps.

The supravaginal septum forms the border between the vesicovaginal space and the vesicocervical space. After dividing the supravaginal septum, one opens the vesicocervical space. Now the lower pole of the bladder can be easily pushed up above the peritoneal reflection in the midline with the index finger. An anterior retractor inserted in the vesicocervical space advances the mobilized lower bladder pole. The peritoneal reflection becomes visible on the anterior wall of the cervix as a tongue-shaped, shiny white membrane (Fig. 118). The vesicocervical space is bordered laterally by the vesicouterine ligament (bladder pillar) in which that portion of the

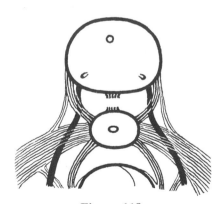

Figure 118.

Vaginal hysterectomy. Separating the lower pole of the bladder. The supravaginal septum is divided and the vesicocervical space is opened. The lower bladder pole is separated upward to the peritoneal reflection, being advanced with a spatula inserted in the vesicocervical space by the right assistant. Laterally, the bladder pillars (ligamentum vesicouterina), coursing from the bladder to the cervix, are stretched. Medially to the bladder pillars at the edge of the cervix are seen the uterine arteries. The diagram above shows the anatomic relationships more clearly.

See illustration on opposite page.

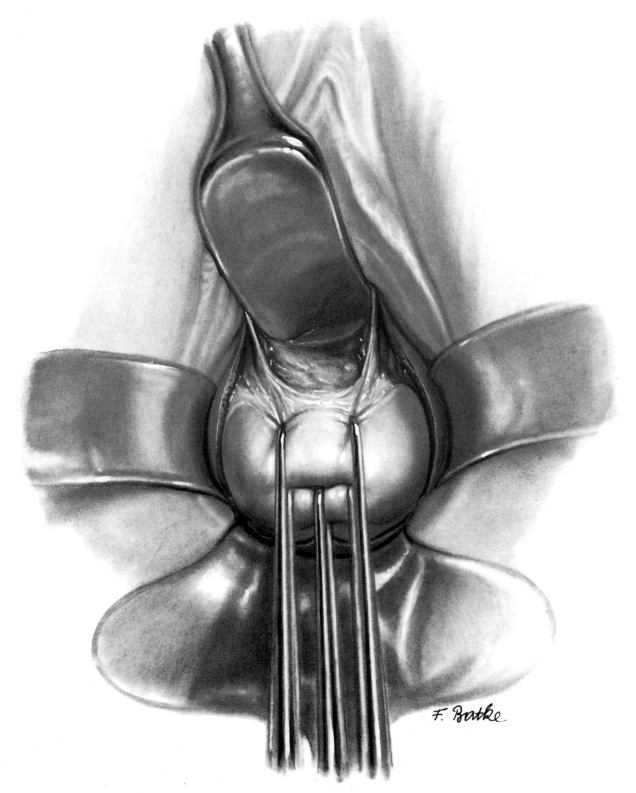

Figure 118. *See legend on opposite page.*

ureter near the bladder courses. In order to avoid endangering the ureter here during later ligation and dissection of the parametria, the surgeon pushes the bladder pillar fibers to the sides bilaterally with his index finger until the ureters are displaced well out of the operative field (Fig. 119).

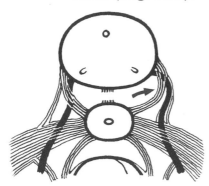

Technical Problems

1. If one severs the supravaginal septum too closely to the cervix, an error often made by the novice for fear of injuring the bladder, then the vesicocervical space will not be reached. Instead one will be probing laboriously in the cervical wall, presuming incorrectly that the faulty planes are the result of a previous infection. This is the lesser of evils. In order to extricate oneself from this maze, one should locate the lower pole of the bladder with a blunt probe inserted into the bladder through the urethra. In this way one will determine if the dissection has come too close to the cervix.

On the other hand, if the supravaginal septum is dissected too near the bladder, the bladder may be injured or even entered. This is easily done and more likely to occur if the lower bladder pole is not pulled up sufficiently with toothed forceps while one is sharply dividing the fibers of the septum.

2. If the assistant elevates the anterior vaginal wall too strongly, the surgeon cannot lift the lower pole of the bladder enough and the fibers of the supravaginal septum are insufficiently stretched.

3. When sharply dissecting the fibers of the supravaginal septum, the fibers may be only partially incised with the scissors. If this occurs and one disregards the remaining connective tissue fibers of the septum that fix the bladder densely to the anterior wall of the cervix, the bladder wall can be damaged when one is bluntly displacing the partially mobilized lower bladder pole with the finger or by increased anterior spatula pressure. Most instances of inadvertant bladder entries occur in this manner.

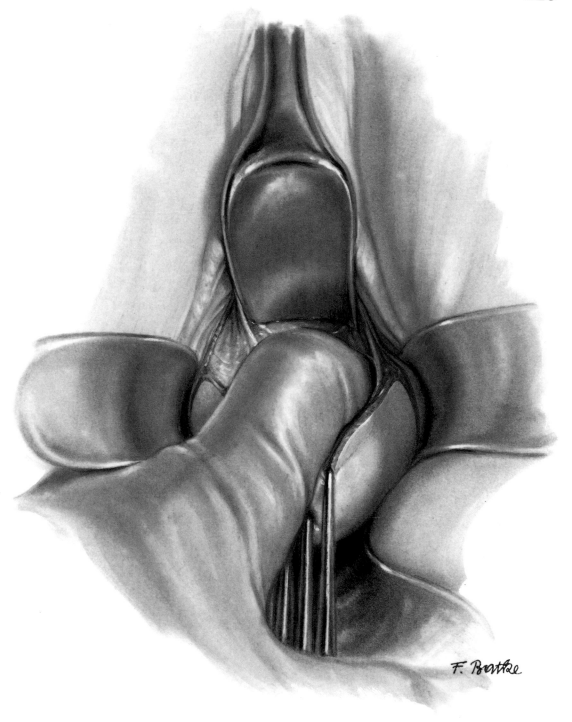

Figure 119.

Vaginal hysterectomy. Advancing the bladder. The bladder is held up by the right assistant with an anterior spatula inserted in the vesicocervical space. The surgeon pushes the fibers of the left bladder pillar laterally with his left index finger, thereby displacing the ureter, which courses in the bladder pillar, out of the operative field. This is shown in the schema opposite.

OPENING THE PERITONEAL CULDESAC

Technique

The uterus is retracted toward the symphysis by the single-toothed tenacula. The posterior circumcision wound gapes as a result of the counterpressure applied on the posterior weighted self-retaining retractor. The surgeon pulls the posterior vaginal wound edge toward himself somewhat with tissue forceps, while pushing the perirectal connective tissue fibers, and the rectum as well, downward with slightly opened dissecting scissors. The midline portion of the incision now gapes widely and the culdesac of Douglas comes into view. Laterally, the tissue fibers of the rectal pillar (ligamentum rectouterina) are recognizable. The operator picks up the peritoneum of the space of Douglas with tissue forceps and opens the culdesac close to the uterus with one transverse cut of the scissors (Fig. 120).

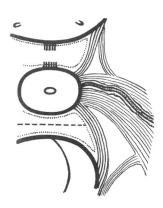

Figure 120.

Vaginal hysterectomy. Opening the culdesac of Douglas. The tenacula on the uterus are pulled upward by the right assistant (the posterior tenaculum has been repositioned to include the posterior vaginal wound edge). The posterior vaginal circumcision wound, which gapes widely as shown, is extended through the fascia vaginalis in the midline to enter the rectovaginal space. The surgeon pulls the rectouterine fold of peritoneum down with toothed tissue forceps to stretch it sagittally; he opens the space of Douglas just above the forceps with a transverse scissor cut, the points of the scissors being directed toward the cervix. The anatomy is illustrated graphically above.

See illustration on opposite page.

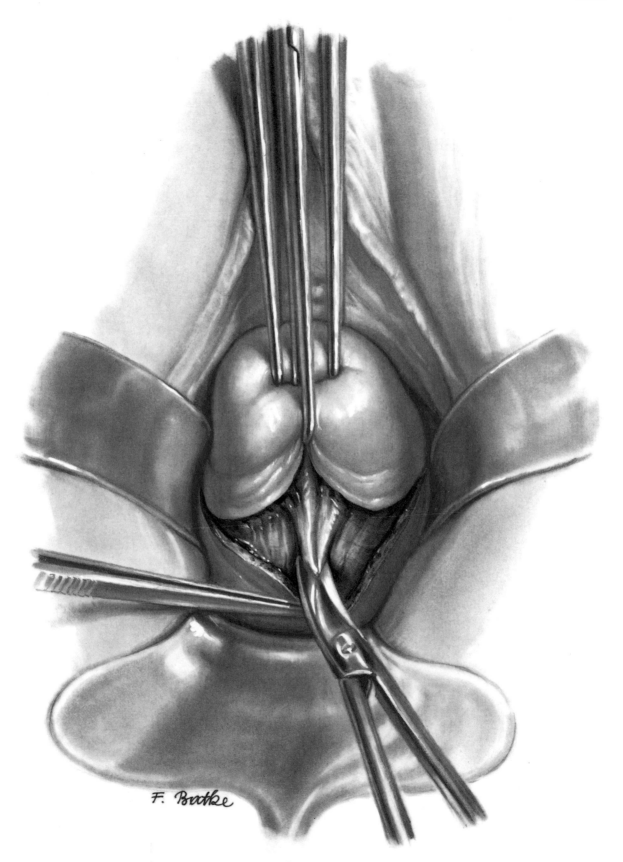

Figure 120. *See legend on opposite page.*

Technical Problems

1. While dissecting the rectum from the posterior vaginal wall and from the cervix, one may approach too closely to the uterus because one fears injuring the rectum. In such an instance the plica rectouterina (posterior peritoneal reflection) is dissected further and further away from the posterior wall of the uterus so that one does not succeed in opening the culdesac because one is operating in the wrong layer. The situation is corrected by grasping the freed plica near the uterus with a toothed clamp, pulling it up, and incising it transversely just caudally to the clamp. In this way one can successfully open the space of Douglas.

2. If the posterior circumcision is not made at the vaginal fornix, but too far cranially in the smooth posterior wall of the portio, the rectovaginal space cannot be opened readily. Here one is dissecting too closely to the uterus as just described and meets difficulty in finding the culdesac.

3. When the posterior vaginal circumcision is carried out too far caudad in the posterior fornix, the rectum may be approached too closely, placing the rectum in danger of injury when the culdesac is opened. This is especially the case if the rectum has not been sufficiently dissected free ahead of time.

4. If the rectum has been displaced from the median aspects of the circumcisional wound and is dissected laterally, it is possible to damage the vessels coursing in the fibers of the rectal pillars.

FIXING THE PERITONEAL CUT EDGE TO THE VAGINAL MUCOSA POSTERIORLY

Technique

The posterior peritoneal wound edge is held tightly in tissue forceps by the surgeon following his incision of the culdesac. The peritoneum is fixed in the midline to the posterior vaginal wound edge with an interrupted catgut suture. The end of the suture is left long

---

Figure 121.

Vaginal hysterectomy. Fixing the posterior peritoneal cut edge to the posterior vaginal wound edge and securing hemostasis. After the culdesac has been opened, the posterior peritoneal edge is sewn to the posterior vaginal wound edge with interrupted catgut sutures. The right assistant pulls the portio upward with the tenacula, while drawing the sutures attached to the posterior peritoneum downward; the left assistant pushes the left vaginal wall aside with a spatula. At the left side, the uppermost corner of the peritoneal opening is being fixed to the vaginal wound edge.

See illustration on opposite page.

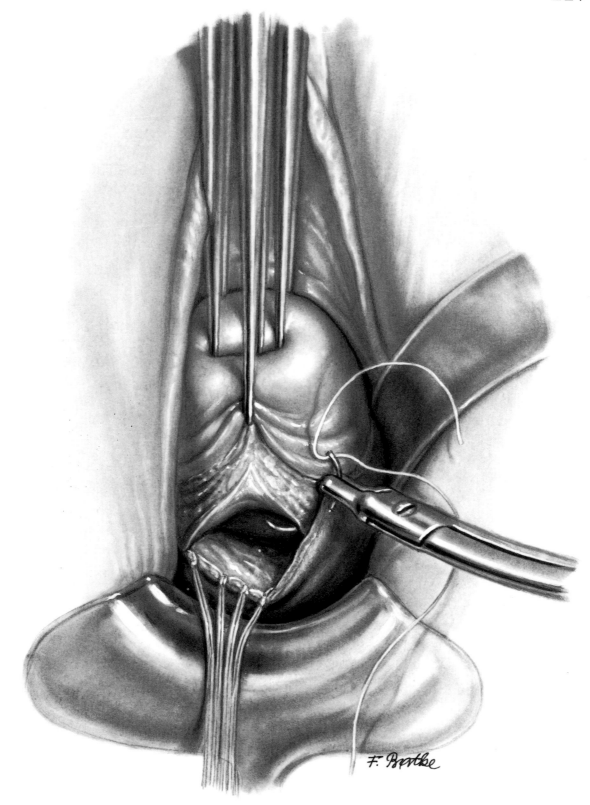

Figure 121. *See legend on opposite page.*

pull upward while the surgeon is pressing the posterior vaginal wall for hemostasis with a sponge forceps applied from outside the posterior cervical wall (Fig. 122), expelling the blood from the peritoneal cavity. Then the assistant once again quickly pulls the ligatures on the posterior vaginal wound edge downward so that the peritoneal cavity gapes open; having thus been cleared of blood, the posterior peritoneal cut edge is exposed and can be further sutured to the posterior vaginal mucosal edge (Fig. 123).

2. Should the peritoneal wound edge not be fixed to the vaginal circumcision edge laterally, bleeding from the vaginal wound edge may be inadequately staunched. This will make later closure of the lateral aspects of the peritoneal cavity very difficult.

3. Excessively strong traction by the assistant on the sutures attached to the posterior vaginal wound edge may tear the delicate peritoneal leaf that is fixed to the vagina.

4. While fixing the posterior peritoneal edge, if the posterior vaginal circumcision wound edge is too deeply ligated, it can lead to injury of the rectum. Danger exists especially when the posterior circumcision is made very far caudally in the posterior fornix so that the rectum is juxtaposed to the vaginal wound edge.

Figure 123.

Vaginal hysterectomy. Additional coaptation of the peritoneal and vaginal wound edges and hemostasis. The right assistant pulls the uterus up by the tenacula and draws the posterior spaced sutures down once again. On the left, the peritoneal edge at the angle of the wound is already sutured to the vaginal edge; this suture is pulled to the left by the left assistant. The posterior peritoneal cavity gapes to show the absence of blood; the cut edge is now fully exposed and can be fixed to the vaginal wound edge.

See illustration on opposite page.

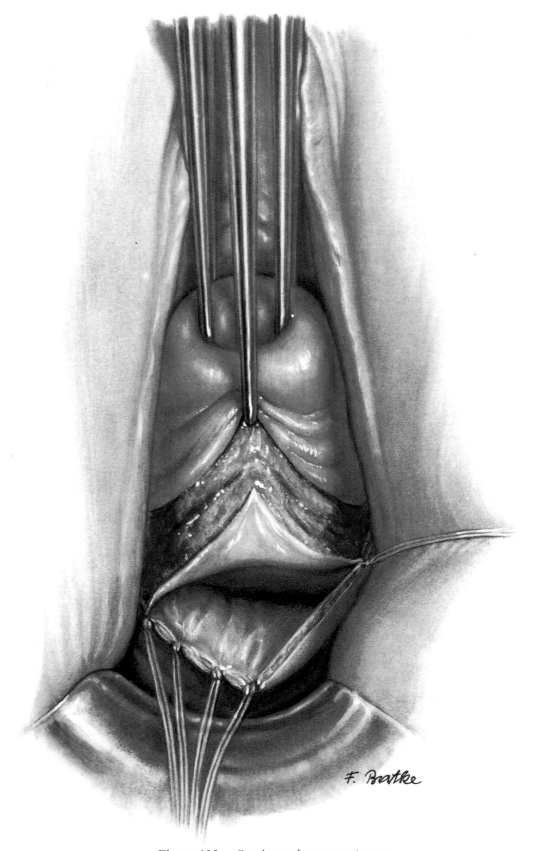

Figure 123. *See legend on opposite page.*

It is important to sever the parametrial bands diagonally about 1 cm. distally to the ligature. Sharply curved scissors are used to make the incision; the scissor points should be directed toward the portio, angulated in to the border of the cervix and parallel to the ligature (Fig. 125). The uppermost medial part of the Mackinrodt ligament, which has not yet been ligated, contains the uterine vessels coursing from the edge of the cervix; it is now ligated with a Deschamps needle (Fig. 127) and the suture is knotted on the preformed parametrial stump. To accomplish this, the surgeon again inserts his left index finger into the opened culdesac, grasping the remaining unligated cephalad portion of the parametrium. He ligates this tissue with catgut on a Deschamps aneurysm needle inserted from the medial side far cranially above the first parametrial suture, but close to the cervix. This second ligature is placed much higher on the edge of the cervix than the first and includes not only the upper aspects of the Mackinrodt ligament but the entire parametrium as well. Before the second ligature is knotted, the clamp on the first suture is drawn to the opposite side and laid over the right lateral spatula to dangle freely.

Figure 125.

Vaginal hysterectomy. Partial division of the left parametrium. The right assistant pulls the uterus down to the right with the tenacula and elevates the bladder up and right with the anterior spatula; the left assistant pulls the posterior vaginal wound edge down by the attached sutures and retracts the left vaginal wall laterally with the spatula. The uterosacral ligament and part of the Mackinrodt ligament are ligated by the first ligature which has been anchored firmly in the lateral groove of the vaginal circumcision wound. The ends of the ligatures were left long and placed over the left lateral spatula; care is taken that no traction is placed on this suture. While the parametrium is being divided from the uterus, the tips of the strong, curved scissors point toward the portio; the incision is made diagonally at an angle to the edge of the cervix. A small piece of the portio mucosa is left on the stump to broaden the distal end of the stump and anchor the ligature on the stump still more securely.

See illustration on opposite page.

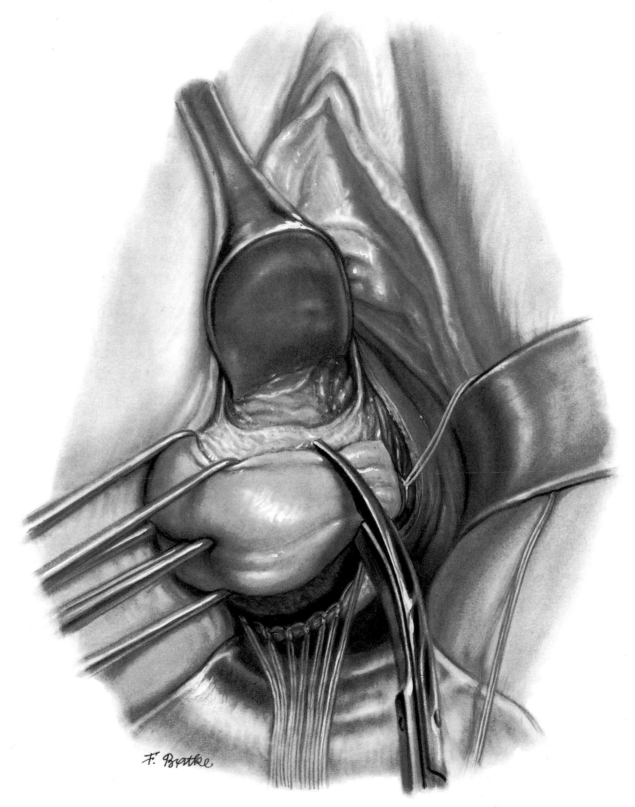

Figure 125. *See legend on opposite page.*

Then the stump of the previously ligated parametrium (which includes part of the lateral parametrium and the uterosacral ligament) is grasped with a long clamp and pulled somewhat downward to the right by the right-side assistant, who exerts moderate force (Fig. 128). The second ligature can now be easily knotted cephalad to the already-placed first ligature. Included in the second parametrial ligature are the uterine vascular pedicle, the entire lateral parametrium and the uterosacral ligament. The second ligature is also left long and is held in a clamp together with the long end of the first suture. Both ligatures are now visually checked by means of the left lateral spatula.

The remaining unresected part of the lateral parametrium, now safely ligated, is transversely resected in the same manner as was done in the formation of the first parametrial stump using the sharply curved scissors. The parametrial tissues are separated from the cervix only up to the point where the uterine vascular bundle becomes visible at the cervical border. The vessels are grasped again with a strong straight clamp before they are dissected free (Fig. 129); they are divided distally to the clamp and ligated with a silk suture (Fig. 130).

The analogous procedure is carried out on the right side to dissect the opposite parametrium. The uterus is retracted downward to the left with tenacula and the bladder is elevated to the left with an anterior spatula. The surgeon inserts his left index finger into the culdesac, grasps the right parametrium and ligates it with a Deschamps needle inserted from above down.

Figure 126.

Vaginal hysterectomy. Incorrectly incising the parametrium. The operativ field is prepared as in Figure 125. Here the scissors are not being held diagonal to the cervix, but parallel to the edge; as a consequence, during the division of th parametrium from the cervix, the upper fibers of the stump are cut short and m; slip out of the ligature.

See illustration on opposite pa

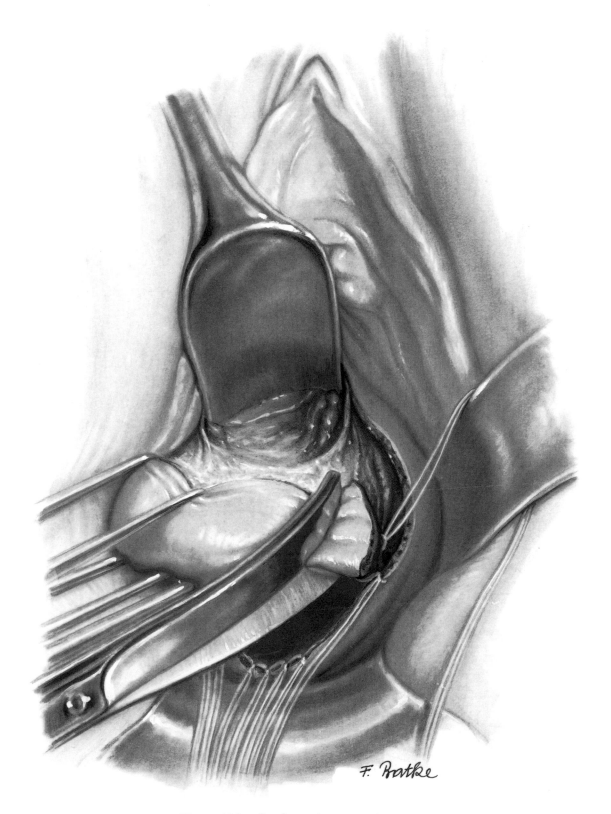

Figure 126. *See legend on opposite page.*

The parametrium can also be resected by the clamp technique instead of ligating it with the aneurysm needle. Strong toothed clamps are placed transversely on the parametrium alongside the cervical border. This approach may be used to advantage when the parametria are very short and rigid.

Moreover, ligation of the parametrial tissue with a strong needle is a rewarding method. But parametrial dissection with clamps plus suture ligation has the disadvantage that sometimes one cannot clamp or ligate high enough on the cervical border. Additionally, the ligation or clamping may be done too closely to the edge of the cervix. It is even possible to suture into the cervical stroma or to catch some of the cervix with the clamp; if this happens, the ligature can slip off. On the other hand, when one ligates the parametrium with the Deschamps needle, the dull tip of the instrument is readily inserted high on the border of the cervix. The needle can be applied closely to the cervical edge if one controls its placement carefully by

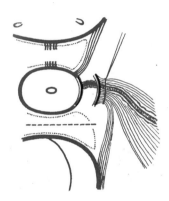

Figure 127.

Vaginal hysterectomy. Ligating the left parametrium; second suture. The right assistant pulls the uterus downward to the right by the tenacula and lifts the bladder to the right with an anterior spatula; the anterior peritoneal reflection is visible. The left assistant pushes the vaginal wall that is situated laterally to the parametrial stump to the left with a spatula. The partially ligated parametrium has been dissected from the cervical border; the long ends of the first suture are hanging freely from the left spatula. The surgeon's left index finger is inserted into the space of Douglas to grasp the cranial part of the cardinal ligament that has not yet been ligated. Using a Deschamps needle, he now ligates the uterine vascular bundle, together with the remaining unligated cardinal ligament as well as the caudal parametrial connective tissue that was previously ligated. These conditions are diagrammed above.

See illustration on opposite page.

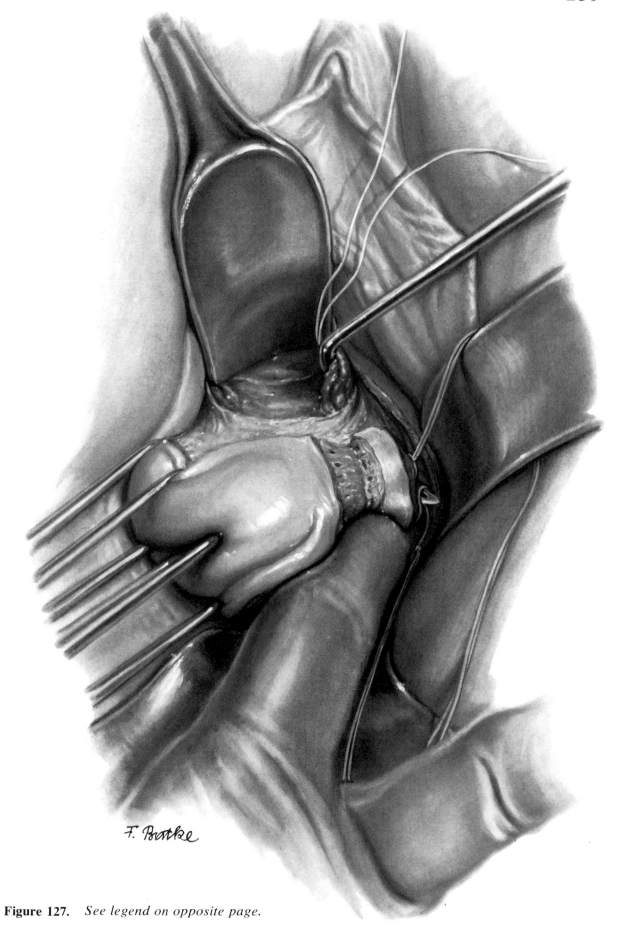

Figure 127. *See legend on opposite page.*

palpation with the left index finger which is inserted into the cul-desac of Douglas against the parametrium. This is a particularly valuable approach, allowing one to ligate as far from the edge of the cervix as desired. Finally, the Deschamps method permits one to ligate the parametria securely above the uterine vascular pedicle, and has the advantage that longer parametrial stumps can be formed. The catgut ligatures applied to these stumps do not come off easily.

Technical Problems

1. If the entire lateral parametrium and uterosacral ligament are jointly ligated with a single suture and resected from the edge of the cervix, the stump may be so thick that parts of it may later slip out of the ligature. Where the parametria are very thick and foreshortened, it is advisable to ligate the uterosacral ligament alone, and perhaps even to suture and divide the lateral parametrium piecemeal before separately ligating the uterine vessels with its own indi-

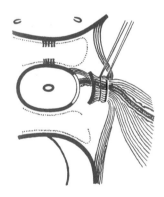

Figure 128.

Vaginal hysterectomy. Anchoring the second parametrial ligature. The thread of the first parametrial ligature is drawn over the tenacula to hang freely over the opposite side. The parametrial stump is grasped with a long toothed clamp and pulled down to the right along with the tenacula on the portio; this is done by the right assistant who uses moderated force. The second parametrial suture is placed and tied cephalad to the first ligature. Included in the second suture are the stump of the previously ligated uterosacral ligament as well as the entire cardinal ligament and the uterine vascular bundle as shown above.

See illustration on opposite page.

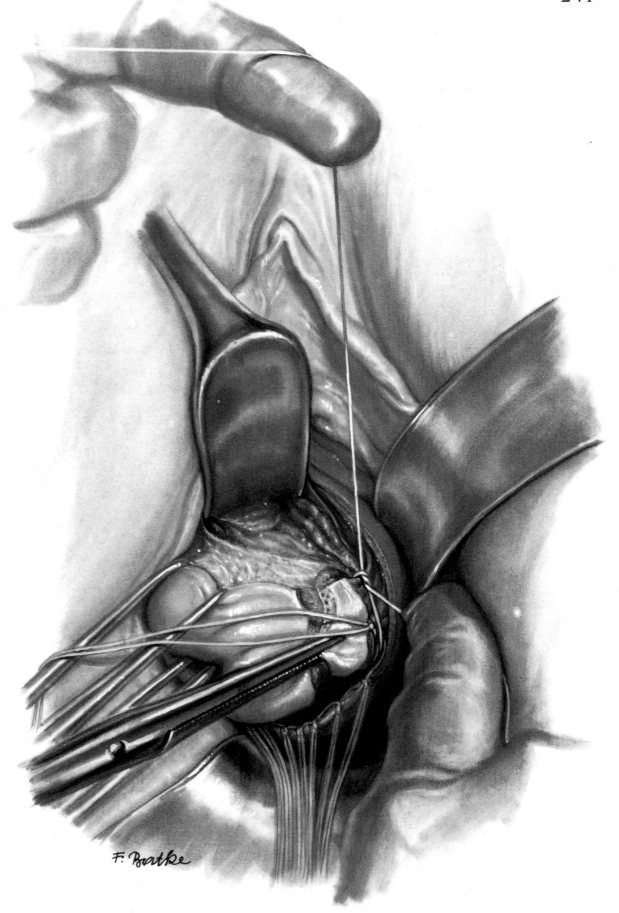

Figure 128.   *See legend on opposite page.*

vidual suture. Ligating too much at a time risks the possibility of the ligature coming off.

2. Should the parametrial tissue bundle be ligated too closely to the cervix, there is great likelihood that the ligature will slip after the parametrium is dissected from the cervix because the stump will probably be too short.

3. If the ligated parametrium is cut transversely, the cephalad aspect of the Mackinrodt ligament stump will be shorter than the more caudad uterosacral ligament stump. This may often cause the ligature to slip away from the stumps.

Other errors that can result in the ligatures slipping off the stumps include the following: (a) The lateral spatula that exerts pressure on the parametrial stump may also press on the ligature. The surgeon should therefore take care that this retractor, when inserted by the assistant to spread the vaginal canal, is placed laterally to the parametrial stump so that only the vaginal wall is gently pushed aside. Similarly, if the assistant pulls the lateral spatula upward too vigorously, it is possible that the stump ligature can come off because the uterus is being retracted downward at the same time by the tenaculum held by the other assistant. (b) With incomplete dissection of the parametria from the cervical edge, the ligature can easily slip from the stumps when the poorly mobilized uterus is rolled forward. This constitutes one of the most commonly made mistakes. (c) While knotting the second cephalad parametrial ligature, if no clamp has been applied to the stump, traction on the first ligature may cause it to come off.

Figure 129.

Vaginal hysterectomy. Dissecting the uterine vessels separately. The uterus is pulled down to the right, the bladder displaced up to the right, and the left vaginal wall is held back from the stump with a lateral spatula. The left parametrium is doubly ligated and dissected from the cervix far enough caudally to expose the uterine pedicle. The unligated vessels are grasped with a short toothed clamp placed transversely to the cervix and divided distally to the clamp.

See illustration on opposite page.

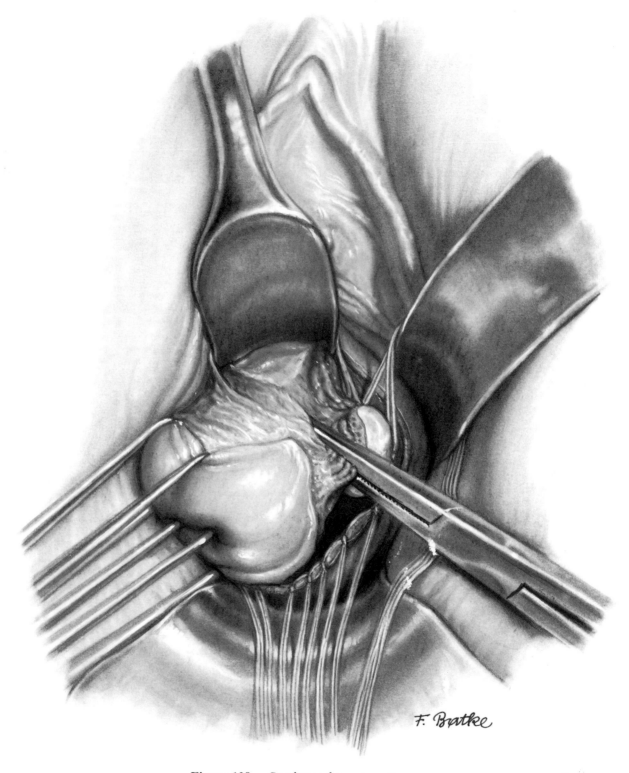

Figure 129. *See legend on opposite page.*

4. During the division of the doubly ligated parametrium from the cervix, one may injure the circumcised posterior vaginal wall with the scissors, endangering the rectum. To avoid this complication, one uses the index finger in the culdesac to ensure that the posterior vaginal edge does not adhere to the posterior cervical wall. If it does, one must push the posterior vagina caudally with the finger. Moreover, during the parametrial separation, the tenacula on the cervical portio should be elevated somewhat in order to be able to visualize the space of Douglas.

5. If the bladder pillar is included during the uterine vascular ligation, the ureter coursing there may be at risk by being pulled very close to the operative field. This complication is avoided by the surgeon pushing the stretched medial fibers of the bladder pillars somewhat to either side with his right index finger; this is done after opening the vesicocervical space and subsequent to dissecting the lower bladder pole. This displaces the ureters laterally and upward so that there is no longer any risk that they will be caught up in or pulled toward the parametrial ligature.

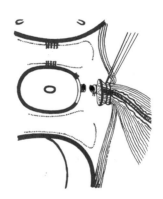

Figure 130.

Vaginal hysterectomy. Ligating the uterine vascular pedicle (third parametrial ligature). The long ends of the first parametrial ligatures are laid over the left lateral spatula; no traction is made on these. The uterine vascular bundle has been divided transversely at the cervical border. The end of the stump, held in a clamp, is turned up by the left assistant's left hand and is ligated by the surgeon with a strong silk suture. The threads of the uterine ligature are immediately cut short. The anatomic conditions are shown schematically above.

See illustration on opposite page.

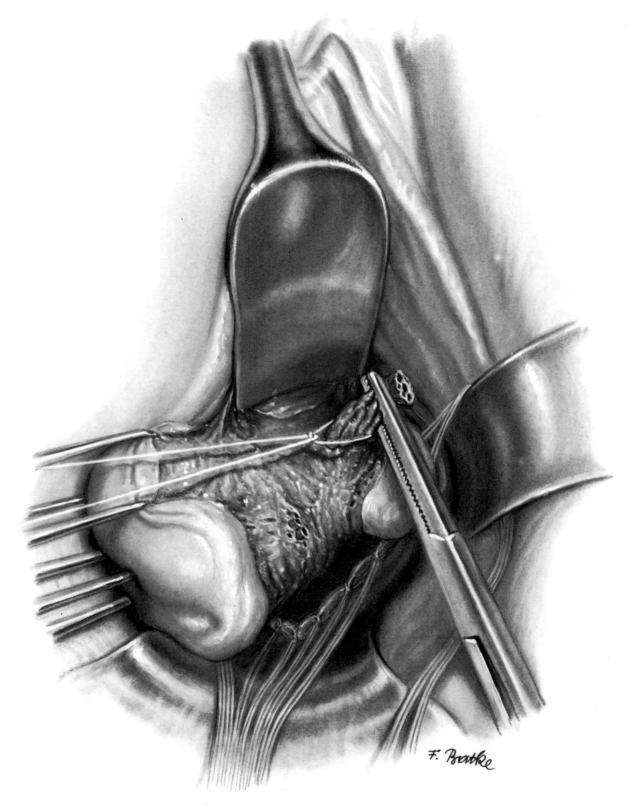

Figure 130. *See legend on opposite page.*

OPENING THE VESICOUTERINE PLICA AND ANTEVERTING THE UTERUS

Technique

The tenaculum on the posterior cervical lip is removed. The uterus is pulled down by the two tenacula attached to the anterior lip. The anterior spatula elevates the bladder in the vesicocervical space. With two lateral spatulas the operative field is exposed. The vesicouterine plica is grasped and lifted with tissue forceps and then incised just caudad to where it is being held, close to the uterus (Fig. 131). If the peritoneal reflection is located high anteriorly because the excavatio vesicouterina is occluded by adhesions from previous surgery or because the bladder peritoneum is fixed to the uterine fundus, the plica can be brought into view by means of a downward pull on a tenaculum placed on the anterior uterine wall.

After opening the anterior peritoneum, the operator places a silk suture at the cut edge (Fig. 132) so that it can be pulled down later

Figure 131.

Vaginal hysterectomy. Opening the vesicouterine plica. The left assistant pulls the uterus down by the tenacula and retracts the left vaginal wall aside with a spatula placed laterally to the parametrial stumps. The right assistant elevates the bladder with a spatula inserted in the vesicocervical space, pushing the right vaginal wall laterally with a spatula placed alongside the parametrial stumps. The parametria are doubly ligated and dissected bilaterally; the long ends of the sutures are draped over the lateral spatulas to hang freely. The sutures on the separately ligated uterine vascular bundles are cut short. At the anterior uterine wall, the anterior peritoneum is visible as a white, shiny, tongue-like structure. The surgeon grasps the peritoneal reflection with toothed tissue forceps, lifts the vesicouterine plica somewhat, and dissects it between the forceps and the uterus.

See illustration on opposite page.

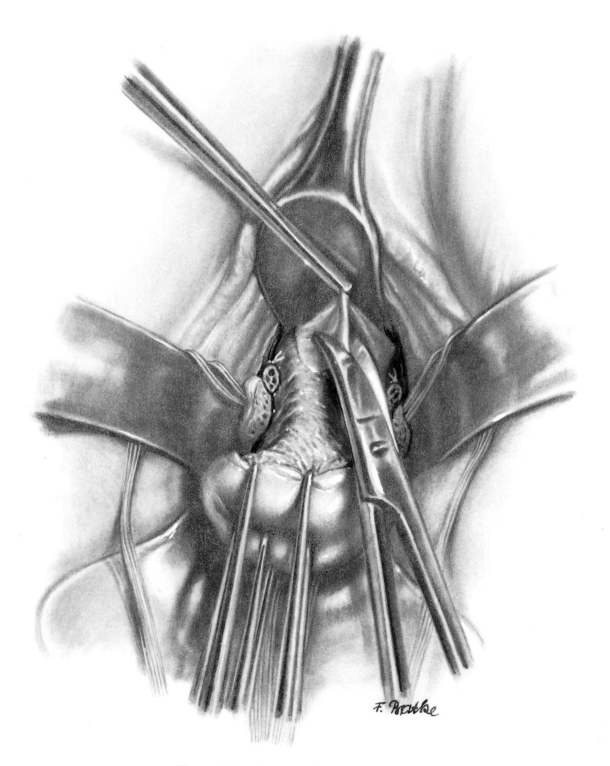

Figure 131. *See legend on opposite page.*

when the peritoneal cavity is being closed. Because there is little space here, he uses a very small round needle.

An anterior retractor is now inserted in the peritoneal cavity to lift the anterior wound edge and the bladder. To prevent the bowel and the omentum from prolapsing, a pack is inserted and the anterior retractor momentarily removed and reinserted to advance the packing strip upward out of the operative field so that the uterus can be rolled forward. For the normally sized uterus, this is successfully done by grasping the anterior uterine wall several times with single-toothed tenacula, progressively climbing upward to the fundus (Fig. 133). As soon as the fundus is reached, the corpus uteri can be displaced by anteversion through the peritoneal opening by a downward pull while the anterior retractor strongly pushes the bladder and the anterior peritoneal wound edge upward. If the uterus is somewhat enlarged, one can facilitate the uterine anteversion by simultaneously pushing the cervix posteriorly into the pelvic cavity by means of the tenacula attached to it.

Technical Problems

1. When the anterior peritoneal reflection is sought too far caudally, one dissects into the anterior cervical wall and is deluded into believing that dense adhesions exist.

2. Earlier in the course of this procedure, if the plica vesico-uterina was insufficiently freed, some bladder tissue may still remain adherent to it; thus, when lifting this tissue with toothed forceps and then dissecting it with scissors, the bladder can be entered. The inadequately dissected bladder pole which is fixed to the anterior wall of the cervix may also be torn by excessive pressure on the an-

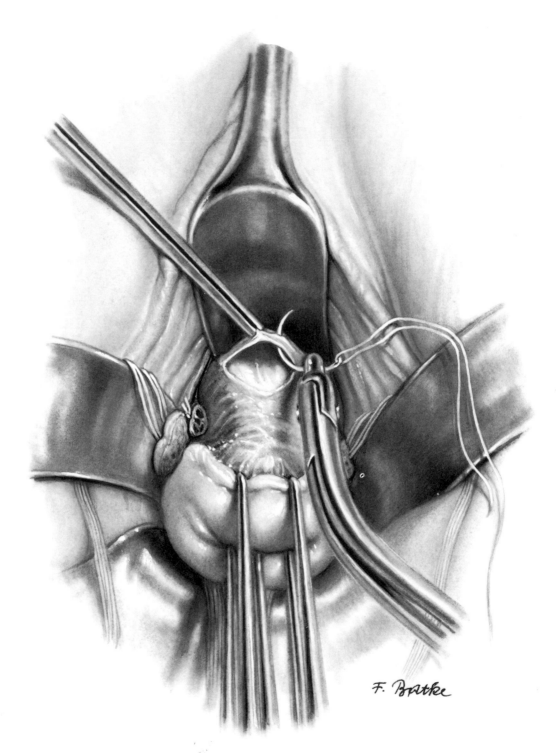

Figure 132.

Vaginal hysterectomy. Suturing the anterior peritoneal cut edge. The anterior peritoneal wound edge is held tightly with a toothed forceps and a fine silk suture is placed with a small, delicate needle for traction purposes.

terior spatula. Therefore, when there is doubt as to whether or not the tissue held in the forceps is peritoneal reflection or lower bladder pole, one should sound the bladder to locate the lower edge of the bladder from the inside.

3. If the silk suture at the anterior peritoneal wound edge is placed with too large a needle, the tissues may be damaged by rough handling because of the limited space available here, and the suture may tear out of the peritoneum.

4. If the silk suture is too heavy, the peritoneal cut edge will tear at the slightest tug, especially the thin peritoneum of an obese woman.

5. When packing the bowel back, the suture attached to the anterior peritoneal edge may tear out or the peritoneum may lacerate laterally, especially if the gauze is inserted without spatula support.

6. The parametrial tissue may be incompletely separated from the cervix so that the uterus is not well mobilized and cannot be anteverted except with difficulty. In addition the parametrial suture may come off as a consequence of the rough handling that will be necessary for the process.

Figure 133.

Vaginal hysterectomy. Anteverting the uterus. The portio is pulled downward by the two tenacula attached to the anterior lip of the cervix; the tenaculum on the posterior lip is removed. An anterior spatula inserted intraperitoneally advances the bladder and loops of bowel together with the anterior peritoneal wound edge. The anterior peritoneal cavity is exposed with two lateral spatulas placed laterally to the parametrial stumps to push the vaginal wall aside. The long ends of the parametrial stumps hang down freely over the lateral spatulas. The uterine ligatures have been cut short. The surgeon places a tenaculum on the anterior uterine wall and pulls the corpus uteri out of the abdominal cavity.

See illustration on opposite page.

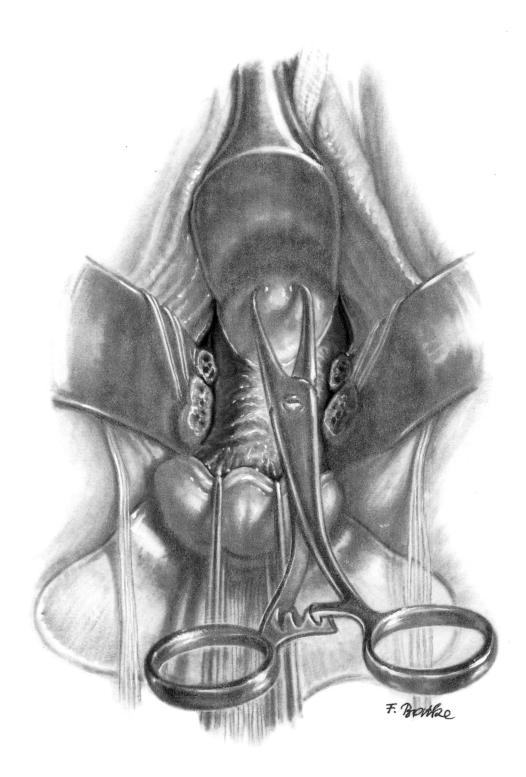

Figure 133.   *See legend on opposite page.*

DIVISION OF THE ADNEXA CLOSE TO THE UTERUS

Technique

In order to dissect the adnexa close to their sites of attachment to the uterus, the anteverted corpus uteri is pulled down to the left by the tenaculum attached to its fundus. The left assistant lifts the packed bowel upward and to the left with a wide anterior retractor. The surgeon checks whether all loops of intestine and the omentum are out of the operative field, and then he places a curved clamp from above on the right utero-ovarian ligament and the tube near the uterus (Fig. 134). He then severs the adnexa between the uterine fundus and the clamp using a pair of strong scissors. A second curved clamp is placed to include the round ligament and the upper part of the ligamentum latum. This permits one to begin to separate the round ligament from the uterus (Fig. 135).

Figure 134.

Vaginal hysterectomy. Dissecting the right adnexa at the uterus; clamping the tube and the utero-ovarian ligament. The uterine fundus is grasped with several tenacula and is rolled forward out of the abdominal cavity. The left assistant pulls the corpus down to the left by the tenacula, turning it somewhat to the right so that the right adnexa are exposed. The left assistant's lateral intraperitoneal spatula pushes the left adnexa back into the abdominal cavity. The right assistant elevates the bowel with an anterior intraperitoneal spatula, while pushing the right round ligament to the side with a lateral spatula. This exposes the site of the adnexal juncture with the uterus. The surgeon places a strong, curved, toothed clamp on the utero-ovarian ligament and the tube; he applies the clamp from above and closes it only after he has assured himself that neither bowel nor omentum has been included.

See illustration on opposite page.

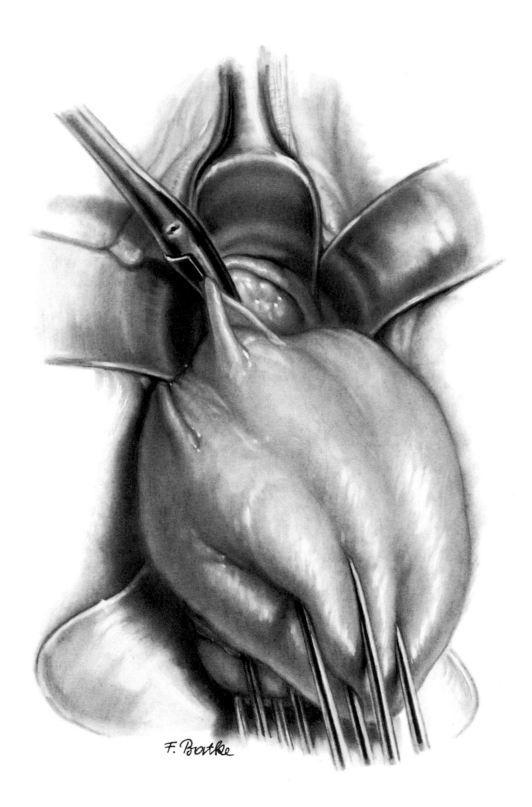

Figure 134. *See legend on opposite page.*

After the right adnexa have been dissected, the uterus remains attached only by the left adnexa. The uterus is quite mobile and can be deflected to the left to provide a good view of the left adnexa and the left broad ligament. The left adnexa can be easily clamped off with one clamp placed from above on the utero-ovarian ligament and the tube and another from above or below on the broad and round ligaments. Then the adnexa are resected and the clamps replaced by strong catgut sutures (Fig. 136); first the uppermost tissues, including the utero-ovarian ligament and the tube, are ligated. The ends of the adnexal stump sutures are left long bilaterally and held in a clamp so that they can be used later for traction when closing the peritoneal cavity.

Technical Problems

1. When placing the first clamp on the adnexa, if only the tube is clamped because it is situated further anteriorly and better exposed, the utero-ovarian ligament is left unclamped.

Figure 135.

Vaginal hysterectomy. Dissecting the right adnexa at the uterus; clamping the round ligament. The anteverted uterine fundus and the portio are pulled down to the left by the left assistant using the tenacula; he also lifts the bladder and the bowel to the left with an anterior intraperitoneal spatula. The tube and the utero-ovarian ligament have already been clamped and divided close to the uterus. This clamp is held by the right assistant who also pushes the vaginal wall aside with a spatula placed laterally to the round ligament. The surgeon grasps the round ligament as well as the remaining undissected part of the ligamentum latum with a second curved clamp applied from below.

See illustration on opposite page.

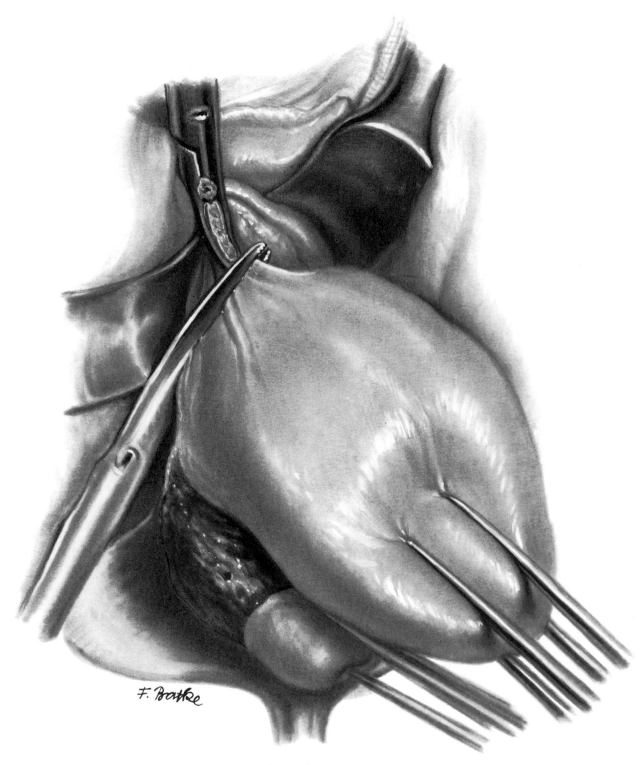

Figure 135. *See legend on opposite page.*

2. If clamps are placed too close to the uterus, the adnexal stumps will be too short and they can slip out of the closed clamp while separating the adnexa from the uterus.

3. Should the tube, utero-ovarian ligament and round ligament be clamped only with a single clamp before division from the uterus, the stump formed is too thick. Part of the adnexal stump can slip out of even a strong, curved clamp.

4. If the second clamp applied on the round ligament incorrectly grasps a portion of the parametrial stump, when the round ligament is severed it is possible for the parametrial suture to be cut. Bleeding will result from parametrial stump vessels.

Figure 136.

Vaginal hysterectomy. Substituting catgut sutures for the clamps. The uterus has been removed; both adnexa are left, having been divided close to the uterus by the clamp technique. The end of the packing that has been inserted intraperitoneally is folded anteriorly over the abdomen. The left assistant pushes the bowel, bladder and left adnexa upward to the left with an anterior intraperitoneal spatula. At the left side, the parametrial and adnexal stumps are visible; the suture ends that have been left long are hung loosely over the left wing of the posterior self-retaining retractor. On the right side, the upper adnexal clamp is replaced by a transfixion suture that ligates the right tube and the utero-ovarian ligament. The right assistant raises the long end of the right adnexal suture and retracts the vaginal wall lying alongside the round ligament with a lateral spatula. In the course of replacing the lower clamp with a catgut suture, one includes and thereby closes any coexisting peritoneal laceration.

See illustration on opposite page.

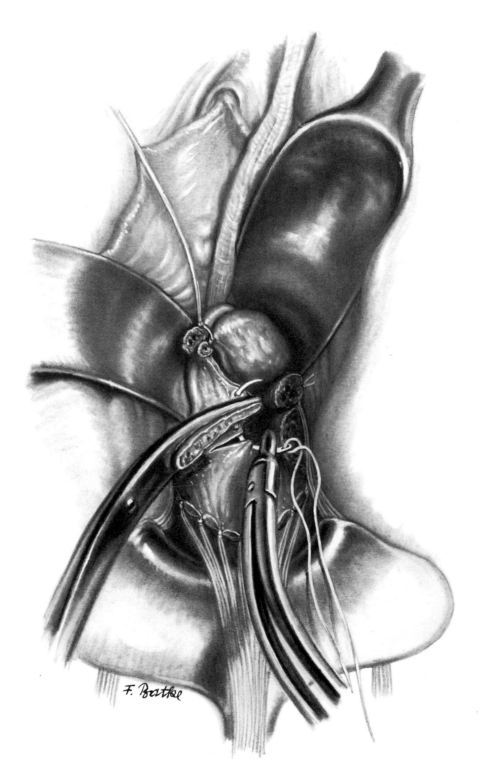

Figure 136. *See legend on opposite side.*

REMOVAL OF THE ADNEXA WITH THE UTERUS

Our usual practice is to resect the adnexa routinely in patients of 48 years of age or older. It is essential for the uterus to be well mobilized and not too large when undertaking to dissect the uterus together with the adnexa, and the adnexa should be free of any pathologic condition. The procedure is begun with removal of the uterus with its adnexa on that side which is most easily accessible.

Ligation and Division of the Right Infundibulopelvic and Round Ligaments

To remove the right adnexa the left assistant pulls the corpus uteri down and to the left while vigorously pushing the bladder upward to the left. In this way the anterior peritoneum is exposed so that the right adnexa come into view. The surgeon reaches down the abdominal end of the tube with tissue forceps and grasps the end of the right tube and the ovary with an ovarian ring forceps, pulling the right adnexa down and left with moderated force. The right assistant pushes the round ligament aside with a lateral spatula to expose the infundibulopelvic ligament. In this way, it can be

Figure 137.

Vaginal hysterectomy. Resecting the adnexa in conjunction with the uterus; first suture of the infundibulopelvic ligament. The left assistant pulls the anteverted corpus uteri forward by the claw tenaculum affixed to the fundus, drawing it down to the left; he also elevates the bladder and loops of bowel up to the left with an anterior spatula inserted intraperitoneally. At the same time, the left adnexa are pushed back into the abdominal cavity. The right assistant pushes the round ligament laterally with a spatula which he holds in his left hand. This exposes the infundibulopelvic ligament. The right tube and ovary are grasped with a fenestrated ovarian forceps. Raising the ring forceps in his left hand so as to lift the adnexa somewhat away from the pelvic wall, he sutures the infundibulopelvic ligament with a Deschamps needle applied from the medial side.

See illustration on opposite page.

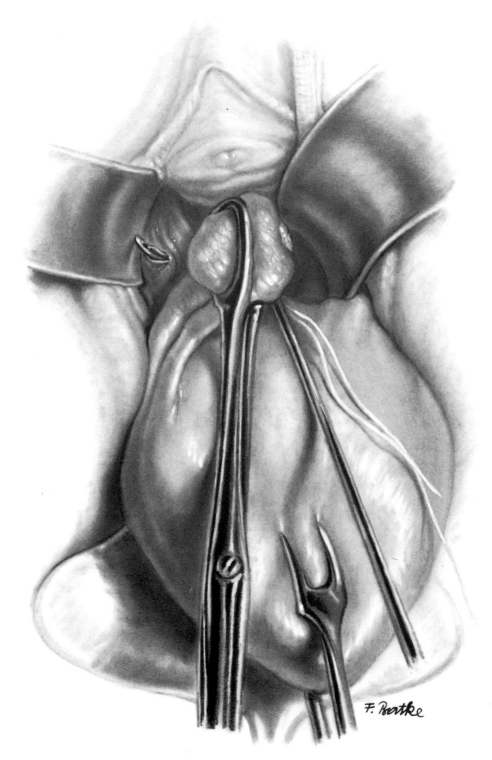

Figure 137. *See legend on opposite page.*

ligated with a Deschamps aneurysm needle about 1 cm. above the abdominal end of the ovary with the suture applied from the medial side (Fig. 137).

The surgeon places the ovarian ring forceps sagittally, lifting the infundibulopelvic ligament a little from the pelvic wall and thereby reducing the risk of injuring the ureter that courses behind it. After the ligation, the ovarian ring forceps are taken by the right assistant. He facilitates access to the infundibulopelvic ligament for the surgeon by holding the handles of the ring forceps horizontally to make much more space available for knotting the catgut sutures. Thus, the surgeon can easily push the ligature up and cinch it with his index finger (Fig. 138). The end of the infundibulopelvic ligament is left long and supplied with a clamp to be used later for traction. To ensure more secure ligation of the large vessels in the infundibulopelvic ligament, another suture should be placed and tied above the first one. This is accomplished if the surgeon pulls the ring forceps as well as the long end of the first ligature down and to the left. Exceptionally, the left assistant may have to do this (see Fig. 97). The infundibulopelvic ligament is ligated once more proximally to the first ligature, with the suture applied from the medial side. Because the ureter courses downward in the immediate vicinity of the infundibulopelvic ligament, it is even more important here during placement of the second ligature to ensure that the ligament will be lifted from the pelvic wall by placing the ovarian ring forceps in the sagittal plane. This second safety suture is cut short so that no one can pull on it. Thus hemostasis of the vessels in the infundibulopelvic ligament is afforded.

Figure 138.

Vaginal hysterectomy. Ligating the infundibulopelvic ligament. The right infundibulopelvic ligament is ligated closely above the ovary. The right assistant's right hand takes the ovarian ring forceps from the surgeon, holding the handles horizontally by placing them flatly against the posterior uterine wall. This gives the surgeon easy access to the infundibulopelvic ligament, providing him with sufficient space in the operative field to tie the first ligature high on the infundibulopelvic ligament without difficulty.

See illustration on opposite page.

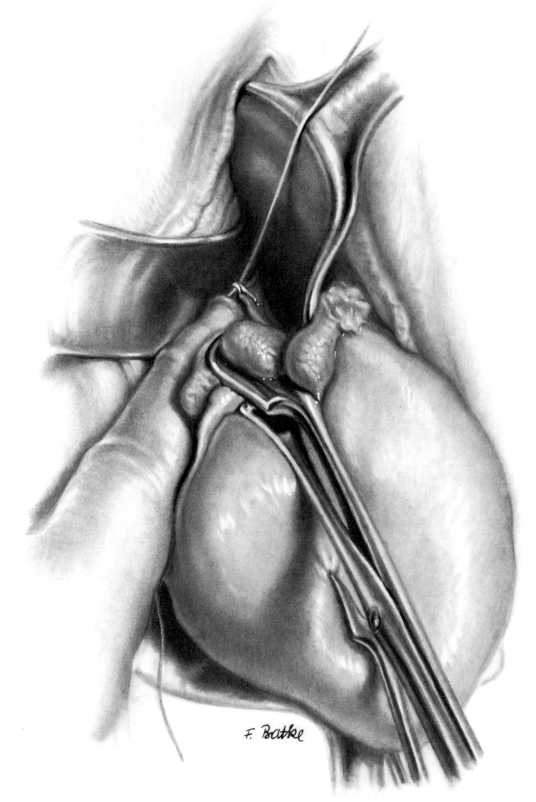

Figure 138. *See legend on opposite page.*

The doubly ligated infundibulopelvic ligament is now divided. Exposure is obtained by the right assistant pulling the first ligature upward to the right, while retracting the round ligament further laterally with the spatula retractor. The surgeon again places the ovarian ring forceps sagittally to lift the ligated infundibulopelvic ligament away from the pelvic wall and severs it between the ovary and the first ligature with scissors. The assistant then releases the round ligament held by his right lateral spatula and repositions the retractor to push only the lateral peritoneal leaf to the side. This permits the operator to ligate the round ligament separately about 1–2 cm. above its attachment to the uterus with a Deschamps aneurysm needle applied from the medial side (Fig. 139). The ends of this suture are also left long and held in a clamp for traction later in the procedure.

Figure 139.

Vaginal hysterectomy. Ligating the round ligament. The infundibulopelvic ligament has already been doubly ligated and divided; the distal end of the ligature was left long, held in a clamp, and folded upward (the proximal second ligature is not seen here; compare with Figure 140). The claw tenaculum on the fundus and the ovarian ring forceps are pulled down to the left and held together by the left assistant, who also lifts the bladder and bowel up to the left. The right assistant has released the round ligament and is now pushing the right vaginal wall laterally with the spatula. The surgeon inserts his left index finger laterally to the round ligament to push the anterior peritoneal leaf of the ligamentum latum sacrally. He ligates the round ligament distally to the infundibulopelvic stump from the medial side.

See illustration on opposite page.

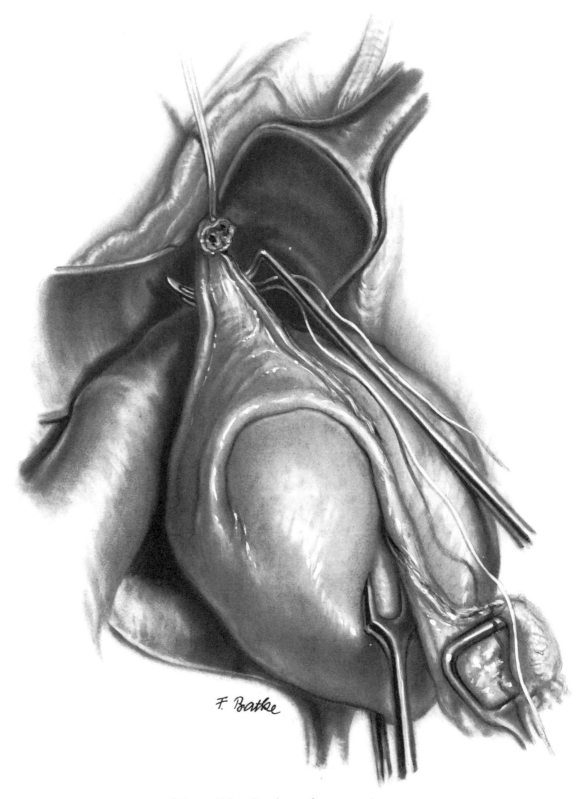

Figure 139. *See legend on opposite page.*

The surgeon can achieve this by directing his assistants well. Only a well exposed peritoneal wound edge can be sutured with exactitude. Help from the assistants is essential (Fig. 143).

One begins by placing half-purse-string sutures at both angles. At the left peritoneal angle, the suture is begun at the anterior peritoneum and one continues to sew from above downward; the right angle suture is begun posteriorly and continued from below moving upward. The needle is always placed into and withdrawn from the inner surface of the peritoneum, progressing clockwise.

Placing the Left Peritoneal Angle Suture and Extraperitonealizing the Stump

While the left angle suture is being executed, the left assistant pulls the left adnexal stump down and pushes the vaginal wound edge and the bladder back above the stump with a lateral spatula. The right assistant pulls the peritoneum of the bladder forward by the suture attached anteriorly, retracting the bladder to the right with an anterior spatula (Fig. 143). The surgeon sutures the anterior

Figure 143.

Vaginal hysterectomy. Preparing the operative field on the left side for closing the peritoneal cavity. The uterus has been removed, but the adnexa were left in situ. The right assistant pulls the traction suture on the anterior peritoneal wound edge upward with his left hand; with an intraperitoneal spatula he lifts the right adnexa and the bladder upward to the right. The left assistant elevates the bladder with a lateral extraperitoneal spatula, while pulling the sutures on the left adnexal and parametrial stumps down and left with his left hand. The surgeon draws the sutures on the posterior vaginal wound edge downward. This exposes the peritoneal wound edge on the left side.

See illustration on opposite page.

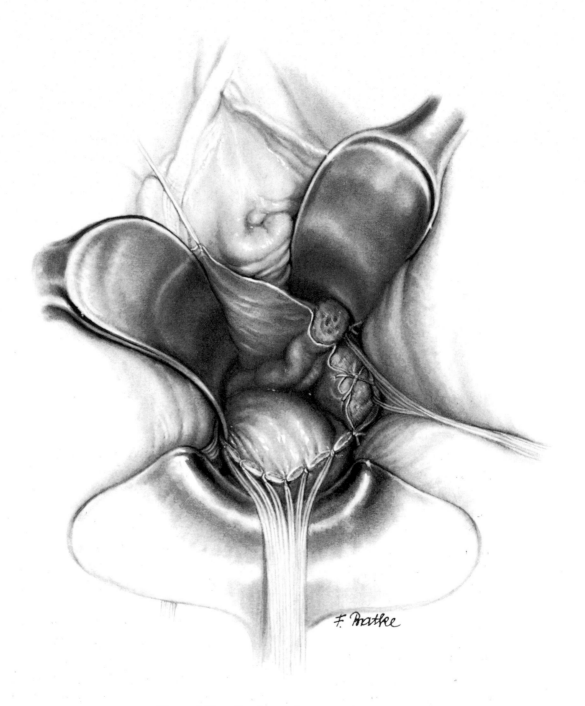

Figure 143. *See legend on opposite page.*

peritoneal wound edge starting from the outside (Fig. 144) and then grasps the peritoneum once again medially to the adnexal stump.

After the anterior and adnexal peritoneal wound edges have been sutured, the right assistant releases the traction suture on the anterior peritoneum and advances the bladder and intestinal loops up and to the right with an anterior intraperitoneal spatula, meanwhile pulling down and right on the several spaced posterior peritoneal sutures. The left assistant changes the direction of pull on the traction sutures on the parametrium and the adnexal stumps so that they are directed upward by his right hand, while at the same time pulling the lateral spatula, now in his left hand, downward in order to push the lateral vaginal wound edge aside.

The surgeon continues placing the peritoneal suture, applying it medially to the parametrial stump and then at the rectal peritoneum where the needle is placed just above the spaced sutures at the posterior vaginal wound edge (Fig. 145). As this half-purse-string suture is being knotted, the left assistant pulls the adnexal and parametrial stumps to the left with moderated strength to displace the stumps extraperitoneally. Then a second peritoneal suture is immediately carried out on the left side to join the anterior peritoneal edge to the peritoneum over the rectum. After the second peritoneal suture is tied, the long ends of the purse-string suture are cut.

Placing the Right Peritoneal Angle Half-Purse-String Suture

The right angle suture is placed in a manner analogous to the technique used on the left, but there is no reversal of direction needed in that the posterior peritoneum is taken up first and the needle is advanced from below up to the anterior peritoneal edge at the bladder. The right assistant pulls the adnexal and parametrial stumps upward to the right and pushes the vaginal wall laterally with a spatula. The left assistant pulls the posterior vaginal sutures down to the left and pushes the bladder and the anterior peritoneum up to the left with an intraperitoneal spatula. The surgeon first sutures the rectal peritoneum just above the posterior vaginal edge; next he stitches the peritoneum medially to the parametrial stump, drawing the needle through the tissues once (Fig. 146).

The right assistant now changes the direction of pull placed on the sutures attached to the parametrial and adnexal stumps, drawing them downward to the right with his right hand; with a spatula in his left hand he elevates the bladder to the right. The surgeon now continues suturing the right peritoneal angle, starting at the parametrium medially to the adnexal stump and ending at the anterior peritoneal cut edge, bringing the needle to the outside (Fig. 147). This

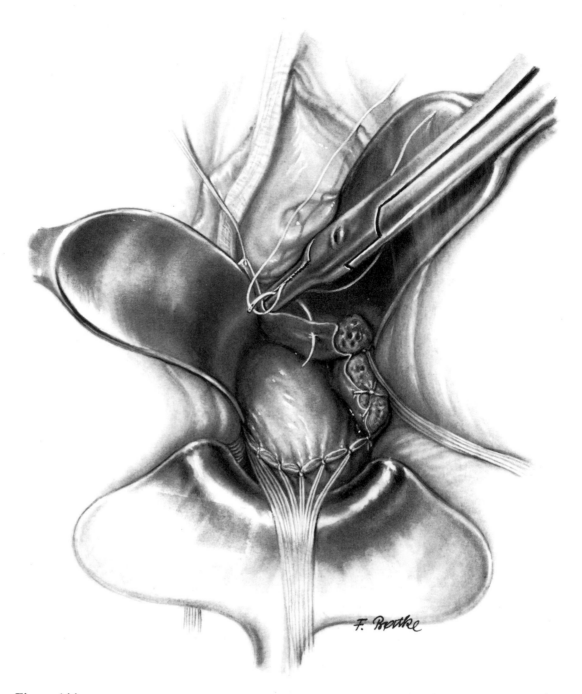

Figure 144.

Vaginal hysterectomy. Beginning the left peritoneal angle suture. The left peritoneal wound edge is exposed as in Figure 143. The surgeon begins the left angle suture at the anterior peritoneal wound edge, inserting the needle from the outside first and then continuing from above down.

completes the half-purse-string suture on the right side. It can now be tied if the right assistant pulls the stumps aside.

A second peritoneal suture is placed on the right side, apposing the rectal peritoneal edge to the anterior cut edge. After this has been knotted, the long ends of the right angle suture are cut. Then the gauze packing that had been inserted in the peritoneal is removed. The peritoneal cavity is thereby exposed by pulling both lateral peritoneal sutures to the side while the left assistant pulls the anterior peritoneal traction sutures forward and the right assistant lifts the bladder with an extraperitoneal spatula placed anteriorly (Fig. 148). The peritoneal cavity can now be easily closed with interrupted catgut sutures (Fig. 149).

In association with extensive descensus high peritonealization is accomplished by suturing the peritoneum at the dome of the bladder with that over the rectum, rather than fixing the anterior peritoneal wound edge to the peritoneum at the edge of the culdesac of Douglas. More effective in cases of this nature is the practice of closing the space of Douglas by uniting the bladder peritoneum with that of the sigmoid starting high up and extending broadly over a wide area.

Figure 145.

Vaginal hysterectomy. Placing the left peritoneal angle suture. The anterior peritoneal wound edge and the peritoneum overlying the adnexal and parametrial stumps have already been sutured. The right assistant lays the anterior peritoneal traction suture on the patient's abdomen and lifts the adnexa and bowel upward and to the right with a spatula held in his left hand. His right hand pulls the spaced sutures on the posterior vaginal wound edge downward. The left assistant changes hands so that he pulls upward on the long ends of the ligatures on the adnexal and parametrial stumps while retracting the spatula at the lateral vaginal wall with his left hand. The surgeon grasps the posterior peritoneum above the vaginal wound edge with the needle.

See illustration on opposite page.

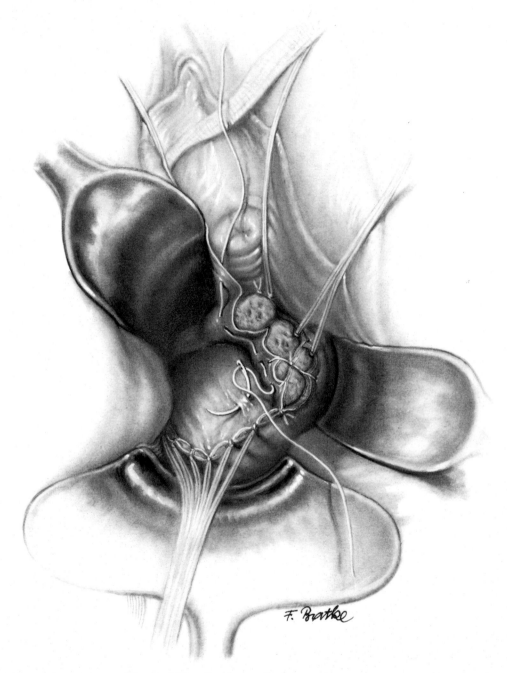

Figure 145.   *See legend on opposite page.*

Technical Problems

1. The adnexal stumps may not be pulled far enough forward during the placement of the angle suture or the medially-adherent peritoneum may not be grasped high enough. If this occurs, a hole is left in the peritoneum after the angle suture has been tied; through it the adnexal stumps can retract to lie intraperitoneally. Since they would no longer be covered by the peritoneum under these conditions, the omentum or a loop of intestine can become adherent and bowel obstruction may result.

2. If the angle suture of the peritoneum is placed too deeply, blood vessels may be punctured and hematomas occur.

3. When the peritoneum is grasped too deeply in the area of the adnexal stumps, the underlying ureter can be kinked or even injured.

4. Should the anterior spatula push the bladder extraperitoneally in too vigorous a manner after the angle suture and the second peritoneal suture have been placed, the anterior edge of the peritoneum disappears upward so that it can be grasped only with difficulty.

5. The catgut sutures used for closing the peritoneal cavity, if too thick, will work their way through the tissues and the peritoneum will be torn. It is best to use size 0 chromic catgut for the angle sutures and size 00 chromic catgut for other peritoneal sutures.

Figure 146.

Vaginal hysterectomy. Suturing the right peritoneal angle. The left assistant pulls down on the spaced sutures affixed to the posterior vaginal wound edge with his left hand, while pushing the left adnexa, bladder and bowel upward to the left with an intraperitoneal spatula. The right assistant retracts the vaginal wound edge to the side with a lateral spatula and lifts the right parametrial and adnexal stumps with his left hand. The right peritoneal wound edge is thus exposed. The surgeon initiates the right peritoneal angle suture at the posterior peritoneum, progressively suturing it from below upward. The posterior peritoneum and the peritoneum overlying the parametrial stump are shown already sutured.

See illustration on opposite page.

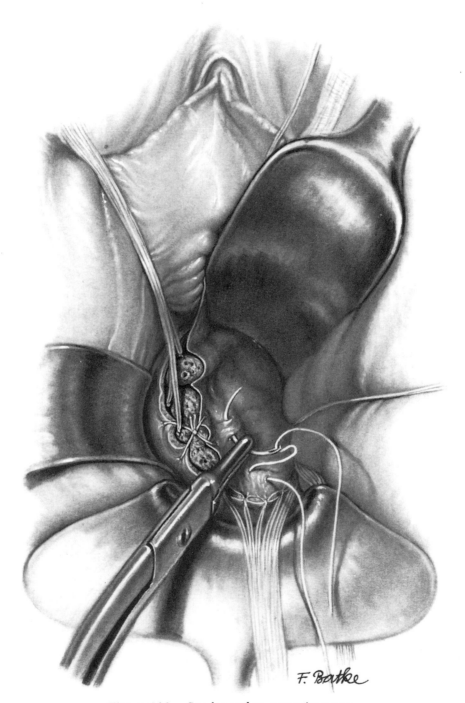

Figure 146.   *See legend on opposite page.*

CARE OF THE VAGINAL STUMPS

After the peritoneal cavity has been carefully closed, the vaginal stump is left wide open to permit drainage of the secretions that are constantly collecting. We merely tamponade the subperitoneal space for 48 hours, allowing the open vaginal cuff to heal by granulation. We prefer to refrain from joining the adnexal stumps transversely in the midline because we are not convinced that this practice prevents descent of the vaginal culdesac. This opinion is reinforced by the fact that fixing the stumps to the vaginal cuff in the course of performing many abdominal hysterectomies in patients with descensus vaginae did not prevent further descent of the vagina. More often we suture the cardinal and uterosacral ligaments laterally into the vaginal circumcision wound causing the vagina to be placed on stretch. It is our opinion that it would also be advantageous to unite these fixed corners of the vaginal cuff medially as well.

Figure 147.

Vaginal hysterectomy. Completing the right peritoneal angle suture. The right assistant has changed hands so that he pulls down on the ligatures attached to the right parametrial and adnexal stumps with his right hand and elevates the bladder with a lateral extraperitoneal spatula. The left assistant has also changed hands. He allows the ligatures on the posterior vaginal wound edge to hang down freely, while lifting the silk traction sutures on the anterior peritoneal cut edge as well as the bladder and bowel upward and to the left with an intraperitoneal spatula. The posterior peritoneum and that over the medial aspect of the parametrial and adnexal stumps have been sewn. The surgeon completes the angle suture at the anterior peritoneal edge, suturing from the inside outward.

See illustration on opposite page.

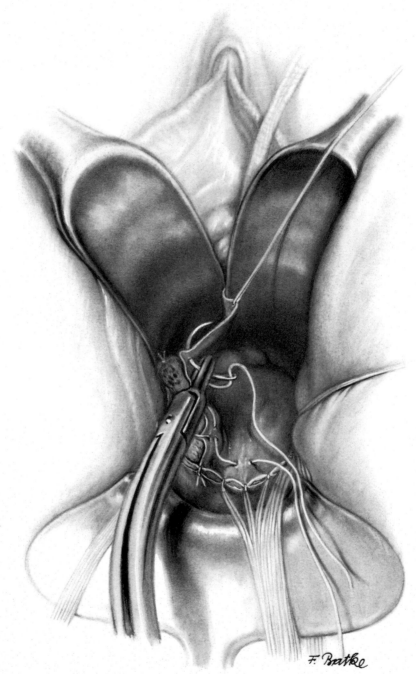

Figure 147. *See legend on opposite page.*

Usually, no bleeding occurs from the vaginal circumcision wound edges when the circumcision of the portio is done correctly by not incising the lateral part too deeply, thus avoiding entry into the veins coursing in the lateral vaginal fascia. Furthermore, the posterior vaginal wound is made hemostatic by fixing the posterior peritoneal cut edge to the posterior vaginal circumcision edge. Should bleeding occur from the anterior vaginal wound edge, pressure sutures are indicated to unite the lateral wound angles of the vaginal cuff. In most cases suturing the lateral angles is not needed to achieve perfect hemostasis because as a rule the hysterectomy is followed by an anterior colporrhaphy which is accompanied by resection of the surplus vaginal mucosa, a step that eliminates the anterior edge of the vaginal circumcision wound. In addition, hemostasis of the midline colpotomy wound and its lowest angle, which corresponds to the lateral aspect of the anterior vaginal circumcision, is accomplished in this way. It is important to leave the vaginal cuff wide open for drainage; the vaginal stump edge either agglutinates by itself a few days after removal of the drainage strip or granulates in after two weeks.

Figure 148.

Vaginal hysterectomy. Closing the peritoneal cavity. The peritoneal angle sutures are tied bilaterally, displacing the adnexal and parametrial stumps. The packing strip has been removed from the peritoneal cavity. The right assistant pulls the right peritoneal suture laterally with his right hand and pushes the bladder back extraperitoneally with an anterior spatula. The left assistant spreads the peritoneal opening by pulling on the suture attached to the anterior peritoneum as well as on the left peritoneal suture. The surgeon closes the peritoneal cavity by joining the anterior and posterior peritoneal edges with interrupted catgut sutures (one of which is shown in place).

See illustration on opposite page.

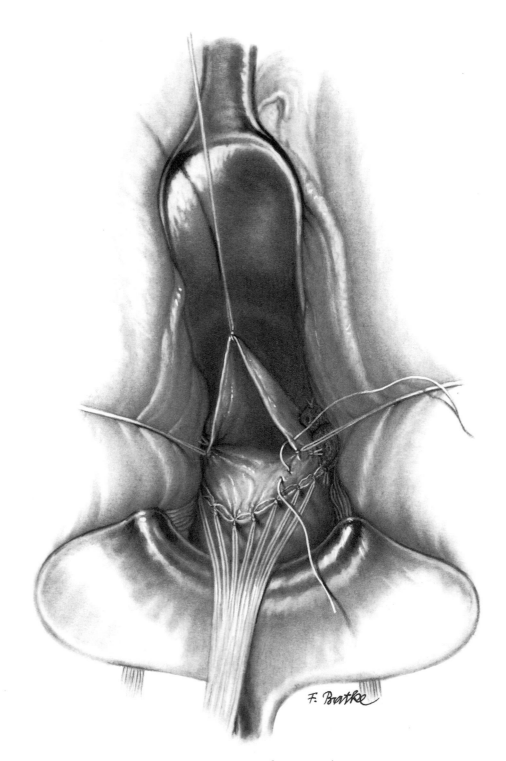

Figure 148. *See legend on opposite page.*

In primary closure of the vaginal cuff by suturing the anterior and posterior wound edges together with interrupted catgut sutures, there is no opportunity given for subperitoneal collections of secretions to drain into the vagina. Moreover, retention of wound secretions can occur above the closed vaginal culdesac, especially in the presence of infection when it may form a subperitoneal abscess that will extend cranially along the path of least resistance into the loose retroperitoneal connective tissue. It gradually becomes palpable as a sense of resistance in the lateral aspect of the lower abdominal wall above the symphysis. Similarly, a retroperitoneal hematoma can develop due to postoperative bleeding from the adnexal stump or the bladder and it may be undetectable because the vaginal cuff was closed primarily. For all these reasons it is important and advantageous to leave the cuff open and to maintain drainage for 48 hours by tamponade. As long as secretions can flow off there is no danger of ascending infection.

Figure 149.

Vaginal hysterectomy. The peritoneal cavity is closed. The vaginal cuff is exposed with four spatulas to show the circular edge of the vaginal circumcision wound as well as the transverse row of peritoneal sutures, the parametrial stumps fixed to the lateral vaginal wound edges, and the extraperitonealized adnexal stumps. Hemostasis is secured at the posterior vaginal wound edge by the spaced interrupted sutures and at the lateral vaginal mucosal edge by the figure-eight parametrial transfixion sutures. In this case, anterior vaginal hemostatic sutures are not placed because an anterior colporrhaphy and bladder plication are to be done for the bladder descent; this will involve extensive resection of the anterior vaginal wound edge. If anterior colporrhaphy were not to be done, it would be advisable to place such hemostatic sutures along the anterior vaginal edge or at least at the corners above the adnexal stumps. The vaginal culdesac is allowed to remain open.

See illustration on opposite page.

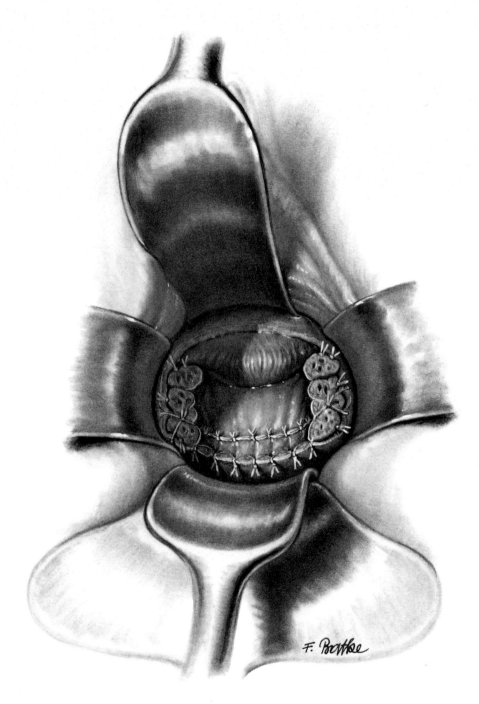

Figure 149. *See legend on opposite page.*

2. Lateral Dissection of the Bladder

After the median colpotomy has been carried down to the proper depth, the bladder is first dissected free on the right side and then analogously freed on the left (Fig. 152). One dissects laterally between the fascia vesicalis and the fascia vaginalis. The technique used is the same as that for the anterior colporrhaphy. However, the vaginal mucosa and fascia together are separated as a single layer from the bladder.

3. Mobilization of the Lower Bladder Pole

To free the lower pole of the bladder, the surgeon lifts the lowermost part of the exposed bladder with toothed tissue forceps and divides the supravaginal septum with several scissor incisions near the cervix (Fig. 153). This opens the vesicocervical space. The lower pole of the bladder can now be advanced bluntly with a finger in the midline to a point above the peritoneal reflection (Fig. 154). Laterally are the tensely stretched bladder pillars.

Figure 153.

Vaginal hysterectomy in total prolapse. Dividing the supravaginal septum. The left assistant's left hand pulls the tenacula down while the right assistant's left hand pulls the upper angle clamp up. Both assistants hold the lateral wound-edge clamps in parallel under slight traction. The bladder is completely freed bilaterally. The bladder neck is exposed. The surgeon lifts the lower pole of the bladder with toothed tissue forceps and severs the supravaginal septum. The tips of the scissors point toward the cervix.

See illustration on opposite page.

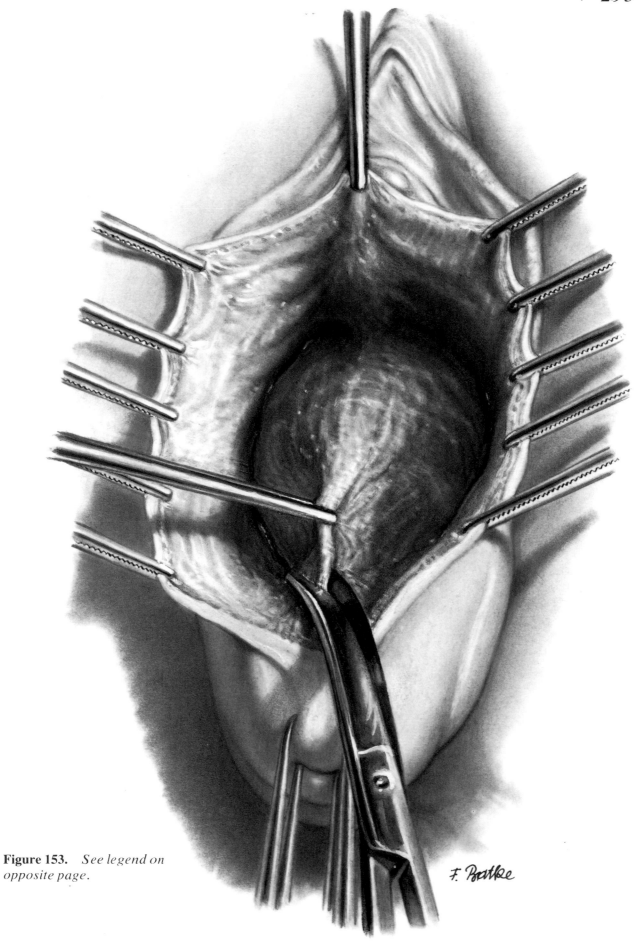

Figure 153. *See legend on opposite page.*

vaginal septum has been dissected and the vesicocervical space has been opened, the surgeon must push the bladder pillars precisely in a lateral direction so that the ureters coursing in them are repositioned out of the area where the parametrial ligatures will be placed. Additionally, in order to avoid injury to the ureter, the stretched lateral parametrium and uterosacral ligament must be ligated and dissected close to the cervix (Fig. 156). The technique for dividing the parametrial tissue bundles corresponds to that of simple vaginal hysterectomy.

7. Uterine Extirpation and Bladder Plication

Removal of the uterus and the adnexa as well as closure of the peritoneal cavity is the same as in the technique for simple vaginal hysterectomy. Plication of the bladder follows along with resection of

Figure 155.

Vaginal hysterectomy in total prolapse. Circumcising the vagina. The bladder has been completely mobilized and the lower bladder pole moved upward after the supravaginal septum was divided. The vaginal circumcision can now be done without risk of bladder injury. Except for those located most caudally, the clamps on the vaginal wound edges have been removed; the assistants pull up on the remaining two clamps. The surgeon pulls down on the cervical tenacula and circumcises the inverted prolapsed vaginal canal with a scalpel. The vaginal circumcision is carried out about 2 cm. cranially to the lowest angle of the colpotomy incision.

See illustration on opposite page.

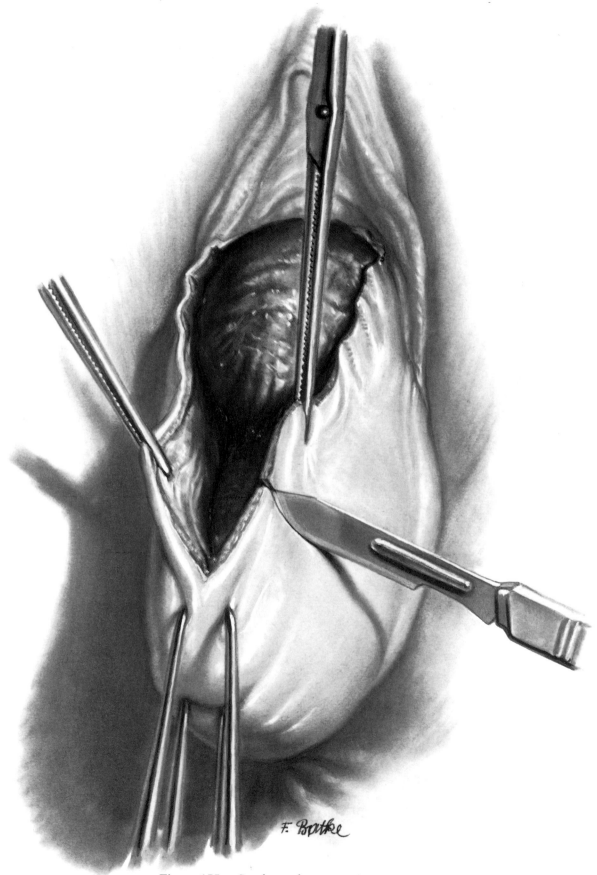

Figure 155. *See legend on opposite page.*

potomy, this can lead to injury of or entry into the bladder in the course of subsequent dissection.

2. After the bladder has been mobilized via a median colpotomy, if its lower pole is not dissected closely enough to the cervix, the bladder wall can be damaged. This hazard is further increased by virtue of the fact that the tissue layers tend to be poorly definable in patients with prolapse.

3. When dissection of the supravaginal septum is not done by a completely sharp technique or the lower bladder pole is advanced above the peritoneal reflection by blunt means, it is possible for the bladder to remain fixed to the cervix, especially if the tissue layers are poorly formed. Under these circumstances, the bladder will be perforated by the surgeon's fingers or by brusque placement of the anterior spatula in the vesicocervical space.

4. Should the parametrial ligatures be placed too high up on the tautly stretched parametria during their ligation, the ureter can be included because it reaches down in this region.

5. Bladder neck plication sutures that reach too far laterally can badly dislocate or even incorporate the ureteral ostia.

Figure 157.

Vaginal hysterectomy in total prolapse. Plicating the bladder. The uterus and the adnexa have been removed; the peritoneal cavity is closed with catgut sutures. The fascial flaps of the vaginal wall are again held bilaterally with toothed clamps which are retracted to the sides to expose the operative field. A posterior spatula provides better visualization by depressing the posterior vaginal wall sacrally. Two purse-string sutures have been placed at the neck of the bladder. The remaining part of the descended bladder has been gathered up with another half-purse-string suture. There is a distinct angulation between the urethra and the plicated bladder neck.

See illustration on opposite page.

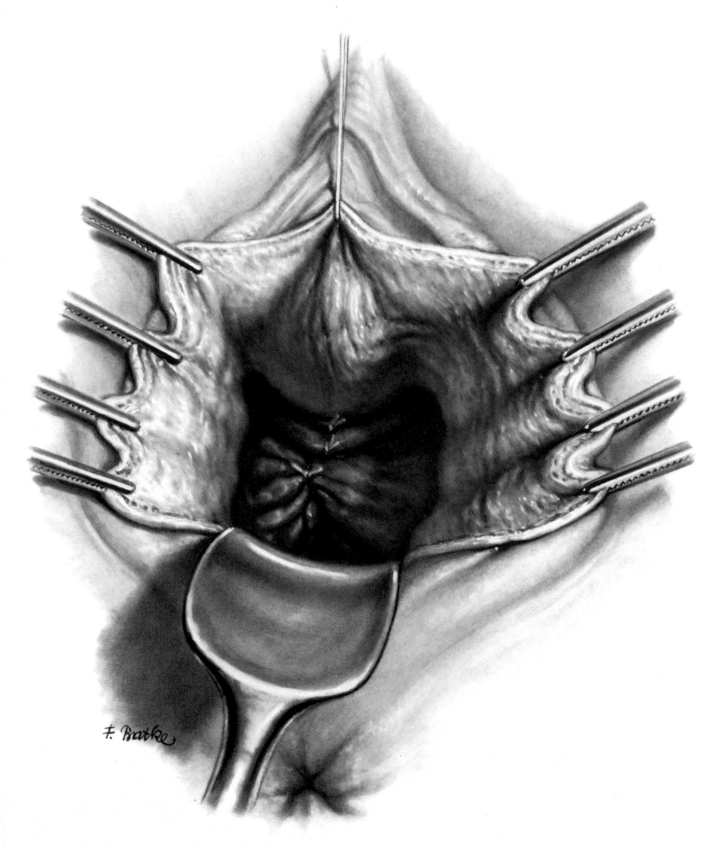

Figure 157. *See legend on opposite page.*

VAGINAL HYSTERECTOMY IN LEIOMYOMATA UTERI

Removing the myomatous uterus vaginally is in the gynecologist's domain, and if done with the right indications, it can work very much to the patient's advantage. The vaginal route can be utilized in both nulliparas and multiparas, provided the distorted uterus fits into the true pelvis and there are no serious adnexal disorders. The enlarged uterus is reduced in size until it can be anteverted out of the abdominal cavity and the adnexal juncture well exposed. There are two procedures available to accomplish this: (a) splitting the anterior and posterior uterine wall in the midline to bisect it and (b) stepwise resection of its tumor masses by morcellation.

Figure 158.

Vaginal hysterectomy in leiomyomata uteri. Bisecting the uterus. The parametria are separated bilaterally and the uterine vascular pedicles are ligated individually with silk sutures. The plica vesicouterina is opened. The right assistant lifts the bladder and the bowel (being held back with a gauze strip) by means of an anterior intraperitoneal spatula. Insertion of the anterior spatula into the peritoneal cavity may be hindered by the coarsely nodular leiomyomata. The anterior cervical lip is held with two single-toothed tenacula. The uterus cannot be rolled forward out of the abdominal cavity because it is enlarged with myomata.

See illustration on opposite page.

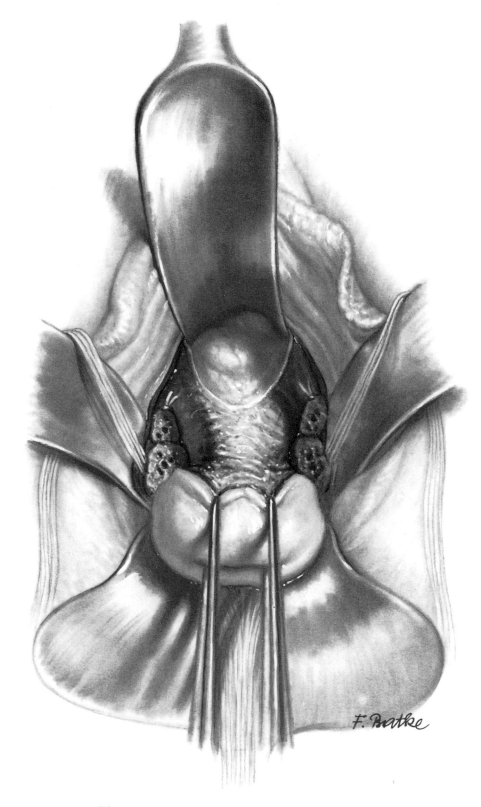

Figure 158.   *See legend on opposite page.*

Bisection is reserved primarily for the uterus enlarged as a consequence of myometrial hyperplasia; the separate halves are readily removed from the abdominal cavity. When the uterus is distorted by multiple myomatous tumor nodules, especially if they are large and located in the anterior wall, successful bisection will be doubtful; under these circumstances, morcellation is more likely to succeed. Both methods can be combined.

The limited utilization of vaginal hysterectomy for the myomatous uterus can be extended with increasing experience and practice. If the organ has good mobility, morcellation allows much larger

Figure 159.

Vaginal hysterectomy in leiomyomata uteri. Bisecting the uterus. The right assistant pushes the bladder upward with a spatula which has been only partially inserted into the peritoneal cavity. Both assistants retract the vaginal walls aside with lateral spatulas placed laterally to the stumps. The threads of the parametrial ligatures were left long and here hang down loosely over the lateral spatulas. The right tenaculum is pulled outward to the right by the surgeon, while the corresponding left tenaculum is pulled out and left by the left assistant. The surgeon splits the anterior cervical wall with strong straight scissors. The first myoma can be seen on the anterior uterine wall.

See illustration on opposite page.

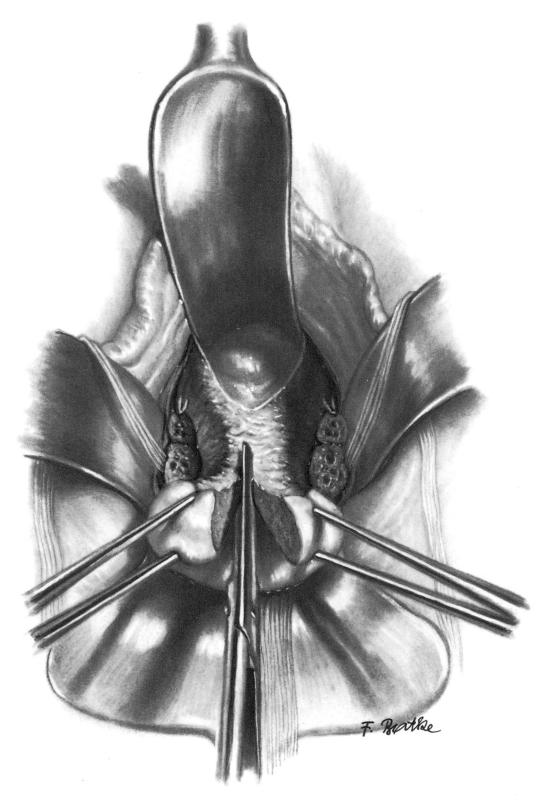

Figure 159.   *See legend on opposite page.*

uteri to be removed by the vaginal route in multiparas. A primary consideration in the vaginal removal of a myomatous uterus, however, is that the morcellation or bisection must always be carried out only under direct vision. In order to achieve this, it must be possible to advance each of the parts to be resected into the true pelvis as one proceeds in stepwise fashion through the operation.

Before uterine reduction can take place, the cervix has to be separated from its parametrial connections to increase its mobility. This can be particularly difficult in cases with deeply seated myomas. Here, one may have to make do first with dissection of the posterior parametrium. After the uterus has been reduced in size and better mobilized, however, one should complete the division of

Figure 160.

Vaginal hysterectomy in leiomyomata uteri. Bisecting the uterus. The anterior cervical wall has been split in the midline. As a result, the uterus becomes somewhat more mobile and can be pulled further out of the abdominal cavity so that the anterior intraperitoneal spatula can be advanced more deeply. At the upper wound angle, the anterior wall of the cervix is again grasped with two additional tenacula that are pulled down by the surgeon and the left assistant, respectively; this permits the lower anterior median uterine wall to be split further upward. The tenacula on the portio are allowed to hang down freely.

See illustration on opposite page.

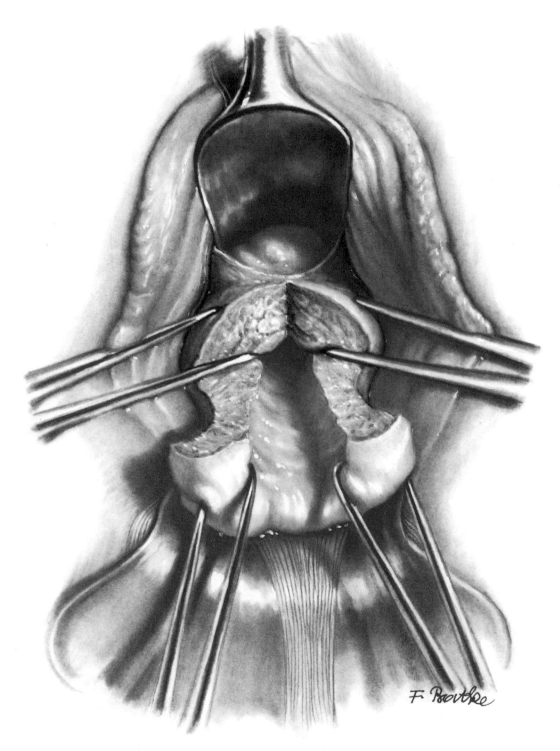

Figure 160.   *See legend on opposite page.*

the parametrium from the cervical border. Moreover, the uterine arteries must be ligated, even before the larger pieces of the uterus are removed by morcellation.

BISECTING THE UTERUS

After the bladder has been dissected, the culdesac of Douglas opened, the parametrium separated from the cervix and the vesico-uterine space opened, the enlarged uterus which cannot be anteverted out of the abdominal cavity may be split in the following manner: The surgeon and the left assistant pull down and out on the single-toothed tenacula that have been placed on the right and left sides of the anterior lip of the cervix. The right assistant lifts the anterior peritoneal wound edge and the bladder with an intraperitoneal spatula; both assistants hold back the labia and the vaginal wall with lateral spatulas (Fig. 158).

Figure 161.

Vaginal hysterectomy in leiomyomata uteri. Bisecting the uterus. The anterior cervix and a part of the wall of the corpus have been split in the midline; the anterior wall cannot be split further at this time because of the uterine size and immobility. The uterus is pulled straight upward by the tenacula on the portio. The right assistant elevates the bladder with an anterior spatula. The posterior vaginal wall is placed on stretch by a self-retaining retractor which also depresses the rectum. The posterior peritoneal cut edge is fixed to the posterior vaginal circumcision wound edge with spaced interrupted sutures; the long ends of these sutures are left to hang down freely over the posterior retractor; they will serve later for traction during reperitonealization. On the posterior cervical wall can be seen the opened culdesac of Douglas reaching down as a tongue-like projection. Therefore, it is now necessary to split the posterior wall of the cervix so as to achieve greater mobilization of the uterus.

See illustration on opposite page.

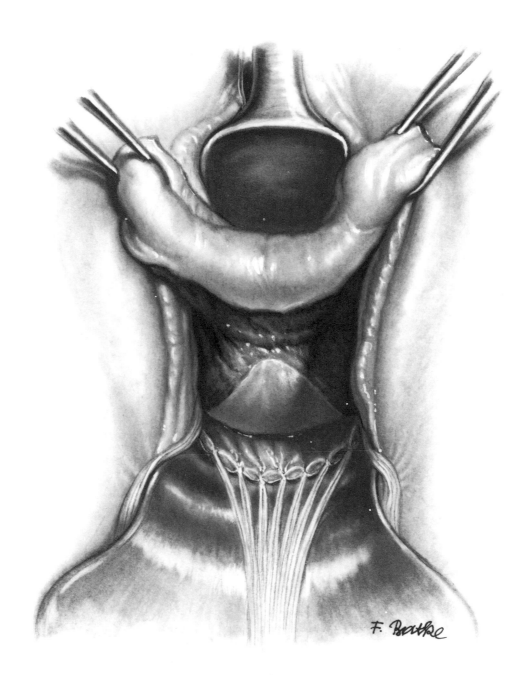

Figure 161. *See legend on opposite page.*

anterior spatula, with which the right assistant pushes strongly upward, can be advanced further and further into the abdominal cavity. The tenacula are placed higher up on the wound edges as the uterus is split as far up to the fundus as possible. One will be surprised how much mobilization is accomplished merely by means of the bisection technique in an enlarged uterus that is split anteriorly but not reduced in size. This phenomenon is explained by the fact that the bisection reduces the anteroposterior diameter of the enlarged uterus, permitting the two halves of the anterior wall to move laterally.

Figure 163.

Vaginal hysterectomy in leiomyomata uteri. Bisecting the uterus. The cervix and part of the posterior uterine wall have been split medially. The two tenacula placed at the cut edge of the cervix together with those on the portio are pulled straight up with moderated force so as to extract the posterior wall of the uterus out of the culdesac of Douglas. The uterus is not yet sufficiently mobile and has to be split further posteriorly. To accomplish this, a second posterior spatula (held in the right assistant's right hand) forcibly depresses the rectum, while the posterior cervical wall tenacula are being vigorously elevated by the surgeon and the left assistant. One can recognize both intramural and submucous myomata.

See illustration on opposite page.

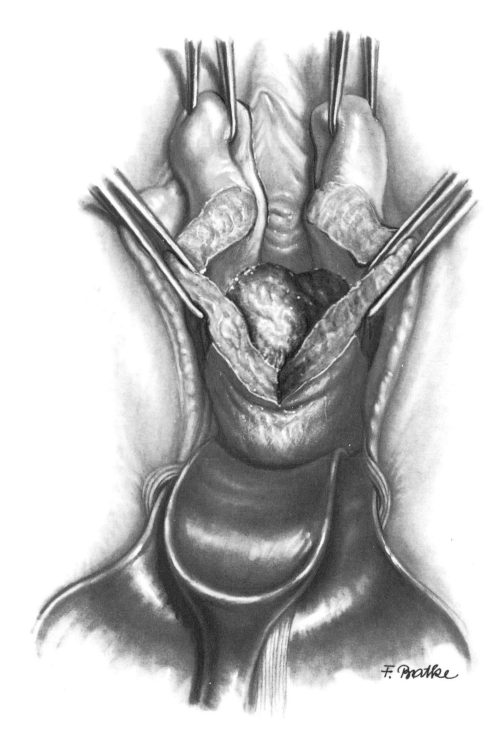

Figure 163. *See legend on opposite page.*

Following this the posterior wall of the uterus is also split in the midline in a stepwise manner with straight scissors. The tenacula at the uppermost wound angle are removed and the uterus is pulled upward by the tenacula attached to the portio (Fig. 161). After the posterior wall has been halved, the corpus uteri slowly descends (Fig. 162); the tenacula repeatedly grasp the apical wound edge so that the midline incision can be extended upward. The wound edge of the posterior circumcision must be pushed toward the sacrum by means of a spatula inserted in the space of Douglas; this retractor simultaneously safeguards the rectum (Fig. 163). The more the bisection progresses, the easier it will be to antevert the corpus uteri out of the culdesac of Douglas. It is often unnecessary to split the

Figure 164.

Vaginal hysterectomy in leiomyomata uteri. Bisecting the uterus. The uterus becomes sufficiently mobilized after the posterior wall has been split so that it is possible to carry the median incision over the fundus to unite the anterior and posterior incisions. The tenacula are moved progressively up to the fundus and the uterus rolled forward out of the abdominal cavity. At the posterior uterine wall, a narrow intact tissue bridge remains to be divided. The surgeon reaches his left index finger behind it to safeguard the bowel, while the right assistant pushes the bladder and bowel upward with an anterior intraperitoneal spatula.

See illustration on opposite page.

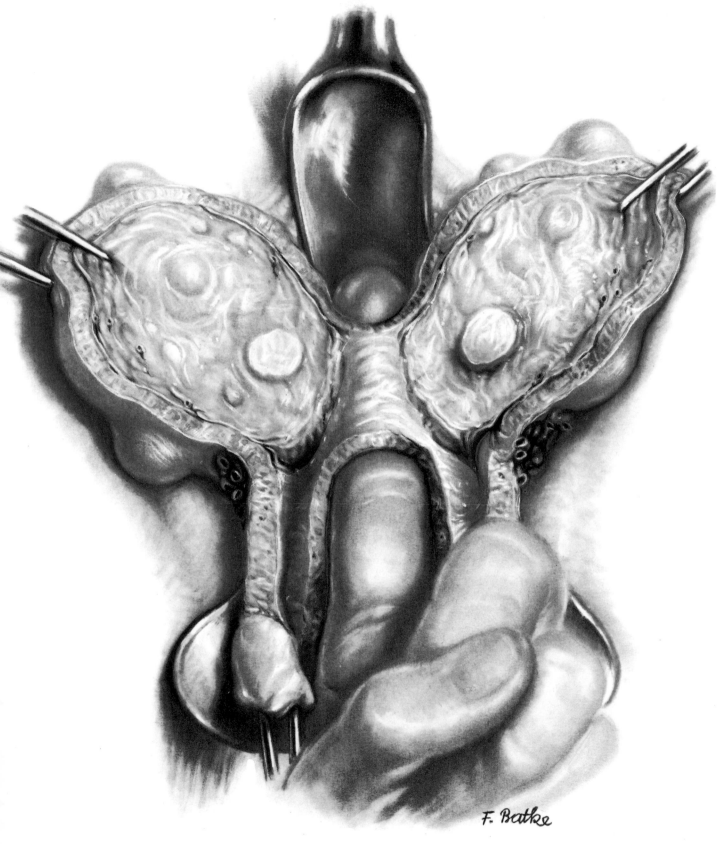

Figure 164. *See legend on opposite page.*

posterior uterine wall up to the fundus because it is possible to pull the corpus out of the abdominal cavity earlier.

The existing tissue bridge still connecting the two halves of the uterus is carefully divided with scissors guarded by the surgeon's index finger (Fig. 164). The tenacula at the fundic halves are now pulled downward, thereby exposing the adnexal attachments to the uterus (Fig. 165). Before the adnexa are separated in the usual manner (Figs. 166 and 167), a wide packing strip is inserted into the abdominal cavity to hold back the bowel.

Figure 165.

Vaginal hysterectomy in leiomyomata uteri. Extirpating the left adnexa. The uterus is entirely split in two and rolled forward out of the abdominal cavity. The right half has already been removed; the long ends of the ligatures on the right adnexa are laid on the right side of the patient's abdomen. The remaining left adnexa are dissected close to the uterus. To do this, the left assistant pulls the tenacula on the portio downward and holds the left labia back with a spatula; the right assistant pulls the corpus uteri down to the right by its attached tenacula. Additionally, the surgeon pulls down on another tenaculum which he places near the insertion of the utero-ovarian ligament. This exposes the juncture with the left adnexa.

See illustration on opposite page.

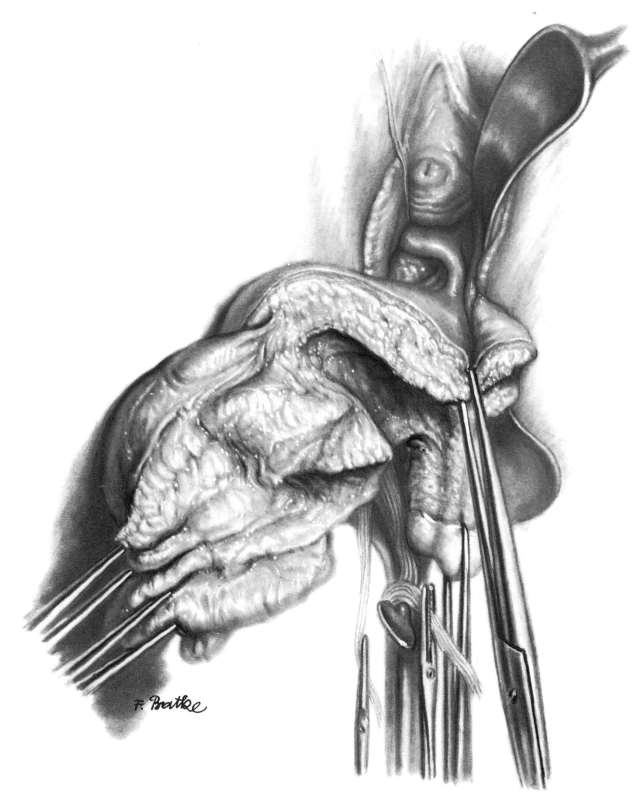

Figure 165. *See legend on opposite page.*

4. Insufficient upward traction on the anterior intraperitoneal spatula increases the difficulty of pulling the corpus uteri out in front of the vulva.

5. If the rectum is not properly safeguarded by a spatula while the posterior wall is being bisected, the rectum may be injured as the midline incision is being extended upward.

6. After the uterus has been bisected and rolled forward, omission of the bowel packing may jeopardize the bowel that may be caught in the clamps applied to the adnexal junctures.

7. The vaginal route should not be persisted in unduly long. As soon as it is determined that the vaginal operation cannot safely be continued (by virtue of adnexal disease, broad adhesions between the uterus and the bowel or omentum, uterine immobility, or underestimated uterine size), one should not hesitate to discontinue this approach (because the indication was wrong) and proceed abdominally.

Figure 167.

Vaginal hysterectomy in leiomyomata uteri. Extirpating the left adnexa. The left tube and utero-ovarian ligament have been divided by the clamp technique close to the uterus. The left half of the uterus is still attached by the round ligament and the remnants of the broad ligament which have yet to be clamped and severed. The surgeon accomplishes this by pulling downward and to the right on the fundal tenacula, which have been relocated forward, and applying another curved clamp from below to grasp the remaining tissues of the broad and the round ligaments.

See illustration on opposite page.

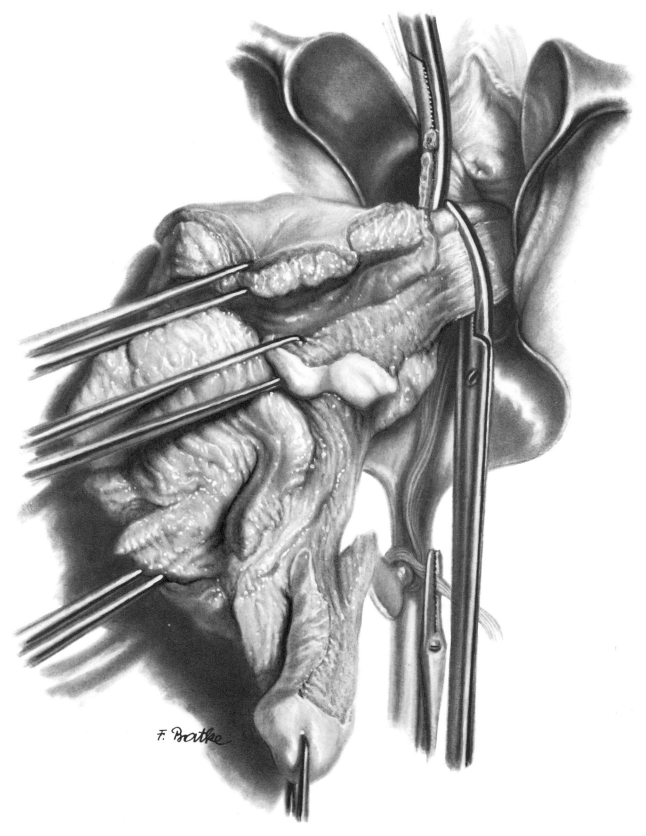

Figure 167. *See legend on opposite page.*

UTERINE MORCELLATION

Vaginal hysterectomy is first begun as already described above: The portio is circumcised, the bladder is dissected, and both the vesicouterine plica and the peritoneum of the culdesac of Douglas are exposed and opened. The parametria and the uterine vascular pedicles are ligated with an aneurysm needle and divided from the border of the cervix. If the operation has been carried out successfully to this point and the enlarged fibroid uterus cannot be rolled forward under the symphysis pubis because of its size, uterine morcellation is in order.

The more accessible part of the uterine wall is first split up to the myoma. The assistants relocate the tenacula up the wall along the incisional edges to bring the higher parts of the uterus down by traction. Small myomatous nodules imbedded in the cervical wall are thus also split with the scissors. Then one grasps the lower pole of the myoma with a single- or double-toothed tenaculum, according to the space available (Fig. 168). The surgeon pulls the tenaculum down with moderated force and cones out the core of the myoma within its capsule in stepwise fashion using a double-edged knife (Fig. 169). This is done while the assistants pull the tenacula on the cervical edges out and down, pushing the labia aside with spatulas. Next, the central components of the myomatous nodules are morcellated away (Fig. 170). After suitable reduction of the size of the myoma, one can dissect the capsule from the uterine wall with curved dissecting scissors (Fig. 171).

Figure 168.

Vaginal hysterectomy in leiomyomata uteri. Morcellation technique. The uterus is split in the midline through the cervix and partly up the posterior uterine wall. An anterior spatula inserted in the peritoneal cavity advances the bladder upward. Further bisection of the uterus is impossible at this time because of the large myomata imbedded in its wall. The myomatous nodules must first be reduced in size by morcellation. The assistants pull the split anterior uterine wall apart by means of the attached tenacula. The surgeon grasps one of the larger submucous myomata with a double-toothed claw tenaculum.

See illustration on opposite page.

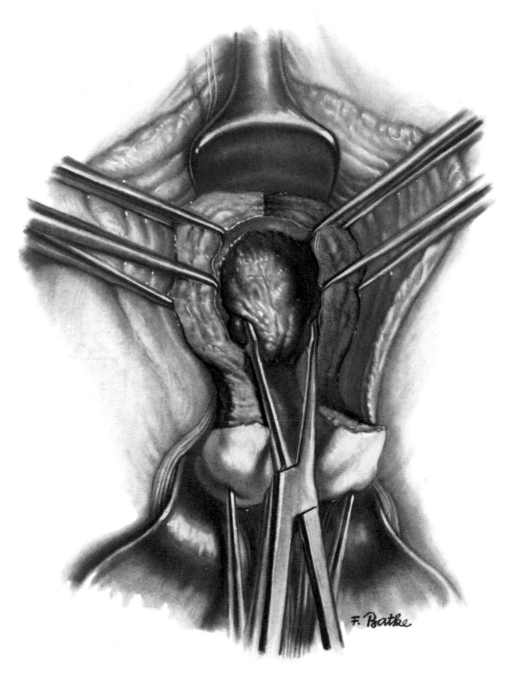

Figure 168.   *See legend on opposite page.*

Intracapsular dissection is not associated with any risk of injury to neighboring organs. If the myoma is very large, one should take care that the uterine wall covering the myoma is split widely to provide as much access as possible to the myoma. As soon as one has achieved some uterine mobility by reducing its size, one pulls the uterus downward strongly, splitting the wall further upward in the midline and moving the tenacula up along the wound edges. Again, the next myomatous core is grasped and cut away with a knife. Enucleation of the rest of this myoma can be done bluntly (Fig. 172). The surgeon pulls the fibroid down with a tenaculum, placing his index finger between the capsule and the surrounding uterine wall to free it. Once the large myomata have been removed, the uterine circumference may be reduced sufficiently to allow one to grasp the fundus with tenacula and roll it out of the abdominal cavity (Fig. 173). The adnexa are divided at their juncture with the uterus in the manner described earlier for vaginal hysterectomy and the peritoneal cavity is closed.

Technical Problems

1. Should the uterine wall covering the myoma not be split widely enough up to the lower pole of the myoma, access for morcellation will be inadequate. However, it is not necessary to split the uterus up to the fundus immediately, but rather to dissect only that section which is accessible.

2. It is dangerous to enucleate a large myoma in toto because one can cut through the uterine wall while sharply dissecting the upper aspect with the double-edged morcellation knife, thereby risking injury to adjacent organs. Moreover, it may be impossible to remove a large myoma by virtue of the immobility of the uterus. It is preferable to excise a number of conical segments in a stepwise manner always under direct vision.

3. If the dissection knife approaches too closely to the uterine wall and is not directed in parallel to the serosal surfaces, it may perforate through the wall and damage neighboring structures.

4. It is important not to be impatient in reducing the size of a large myomatous uterus. One should morcellate small pieces until the uterine mass is small enough to be rolled out of the abdominal cavity.

(Text continued on page 330)

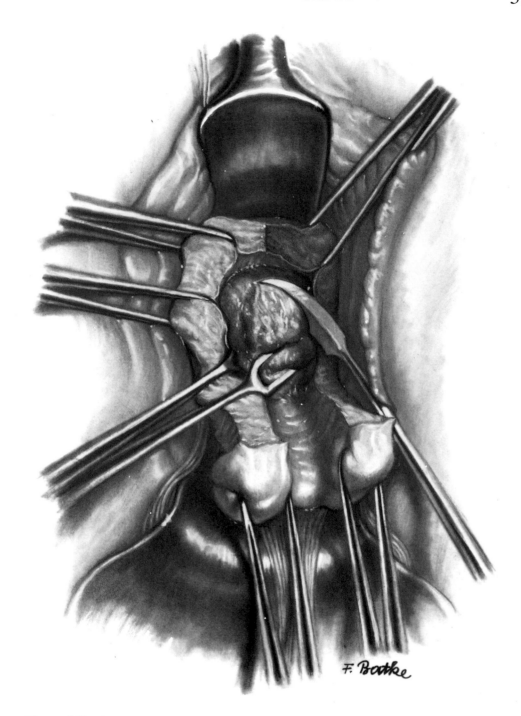

F. Bothe

Figure 169.

   Vaginal hysterectomy in leiomyomata uteri. Morcellation technique. The split uterine wall is spread with tenacula and the portio is pulled downward. The surgeon has grasped one of the larger submucous myomata with a claw tenaculum and is cutting out a piece of it with a special lancet-shaped double-edge knife (note the correct positioning of the knife).

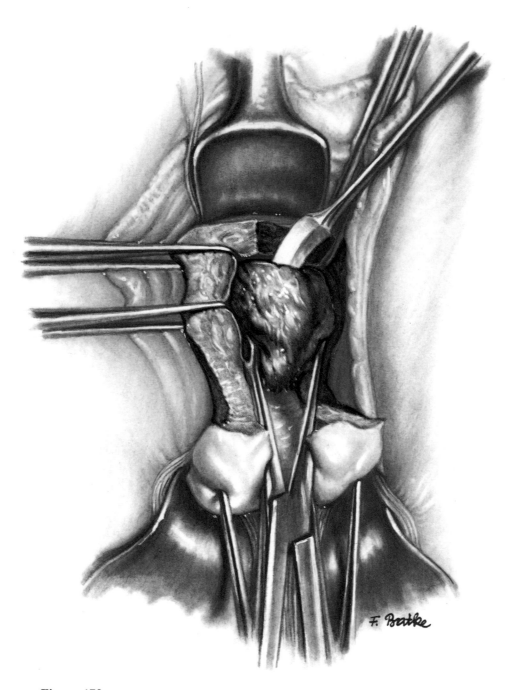

Figure 170.

Vaginal hysterectomy in leiomyomata uteri. Morcellation technique. The operative field is prepared as in Figure 169, but the positioning of the knife here is incorrect. If the knife were to be pushed forward into the myoma, it might perforate the posterior wall of the uterus and injure the bowel.

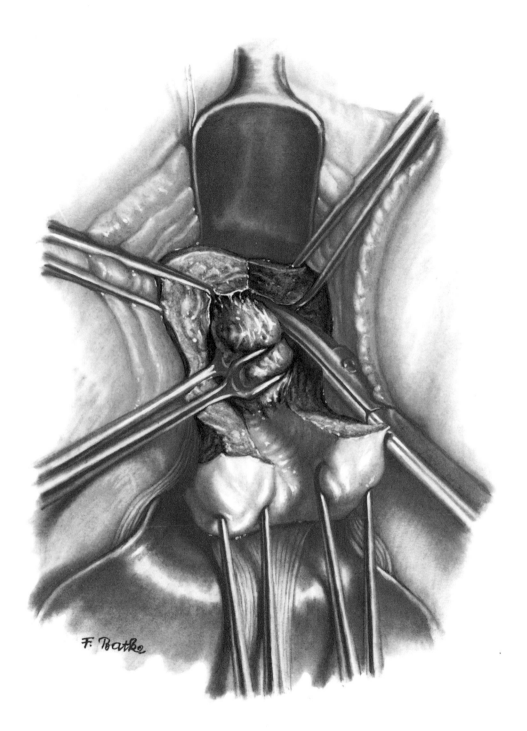

Figure 171.

Vaginal hysterectomy in leiomyomata uteri. Morcellation tech-nique. Having prepared the operative field as in Figure 169, the sur-geon removes a portion of the submucous myoma by morcellation. The rest of the nodule is again grasped with the tenaculum and pulled downward. The uppermost part is mobilized intracapsularly with scissors.

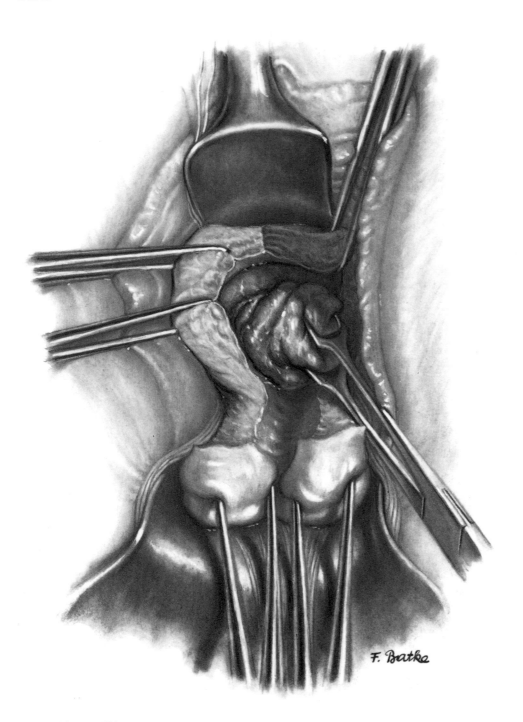

Figure 172.

Vaginal hysterectomy in leiomyomata uteri. Morcellation technique. The anterior wall is then split upward a little more to expose another submucous myoma. This nodule is thoroughly mobilized by intracapsular dissection with scissors so that the surgeon can avulse it with the claw tenaculum.

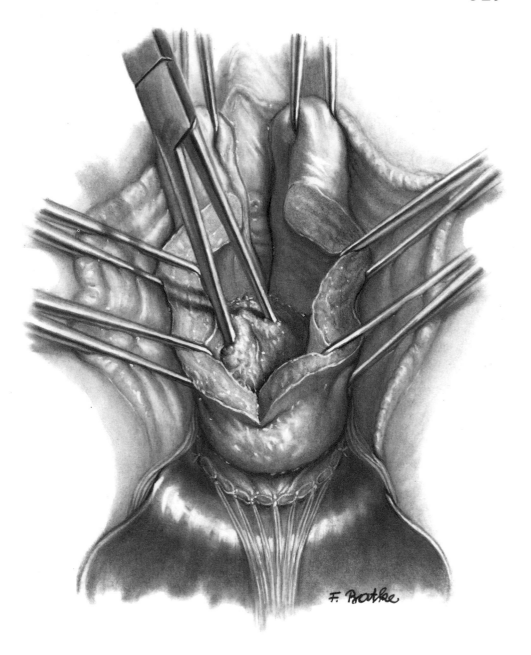

Figure 173.

Vaginal hysterectomy in leiomyomata uteri. Morcellation technique. Several myomata have already been removed. In order to achieve better mobility of the uterus, its posterior wall has also been split medially. When the posterior wall is spread apart, another large myoma is exposed. The surgeon grasps it with a claw tenaculum and pulls it upward so as to morcellate it. In this way the large myomatous uterus is reduced in a step-wise manner until it can at last be rolled forward out of the abdominal cavity.

ANTERIOR COLPORRHAPHY

The anterior vaginoplasty serves for purposes of reconstructing the supporting structures of the bladder floor and the urethra; it is a part of the operative procedure for vaginal prolapse. This operation should always be combined with a colpoperineoplasty, because bringing the levators together where they have come apart provides great mechanical support for elevating the relaxed vaginal wall and correcting resultant urinary incontinence.

Figure 174.

Anterior colporrhaphy. Median colpotomy. The vagina is prepared with two lateral spatulas and one self-retaining posterior retractor. The surgeon pulls the tenacula on the cervix down while the right assistant pushes the inverted vaginal wall strongly upward with the anterior spatula. The median longitudinal incision is begun in the stretched part of the anterior vagina (the incision severs only the mucosa, leaving the underlying fascia intact). The lower wound angle reaches to the transition between the movable vaginal mucosa and the fixed cervical mucosa.

See illustration on opposite page.

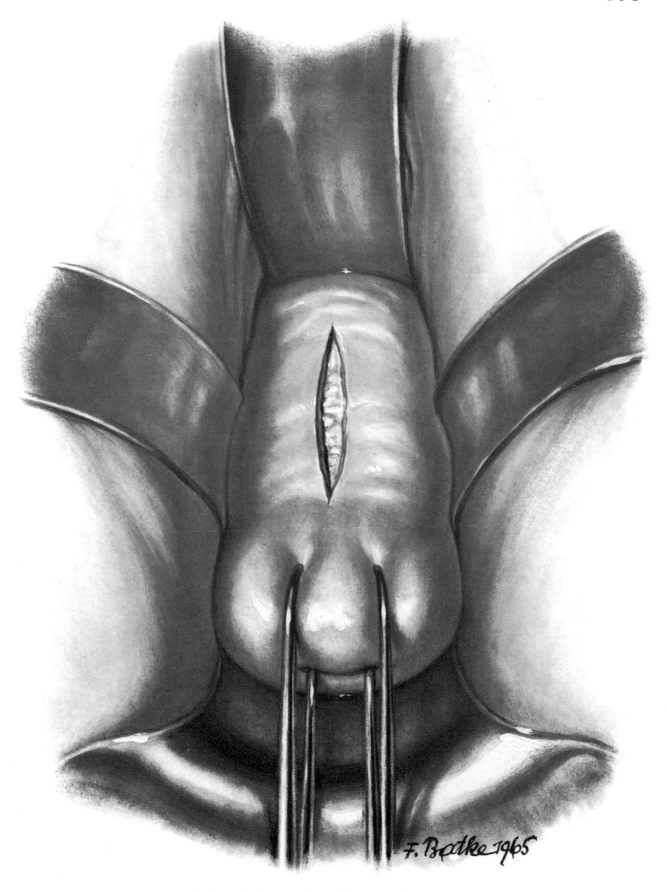

Figure 174. *See legend on opposite page.*

MEDIAN COLPOTOMY

Placing the Incision

A midline lengthwise incision is made in the inverted anterior vaginal wall beginning at the junction of the portio epithelium with the vaginal mucosa and extending to just beneath the urethral meatus. In our opinion, the midline colpotomy incision makes for a simpler dissection of the vaginal mucosa from its fascia or from the bladder than the alternative technique involving the excision of the vaginal wall by means of an elliptical incision.

Figure 175.

Anterior colporrhaphy. Extending the median colpotomy upward. The anterior lip of the cervix is held by two tenacula that are pulled down by the left assistant's left hand. The vaginal wound edges are grasped with two toothed clamps on each side. Those clamps placed most cranially are pulled downward by the assistants in order to stretch the vaginal wound edges further; the other clamps are allowed to hang down freely. Additionally, the right assistant places the anterior vaginal wall on more stretch with upward pressure on the anterior spatula. The median colpotomy has been carried down to the intact vaginal fascia in which veins are visible. The midline incision is extended upward.

See illustration on opposite page.

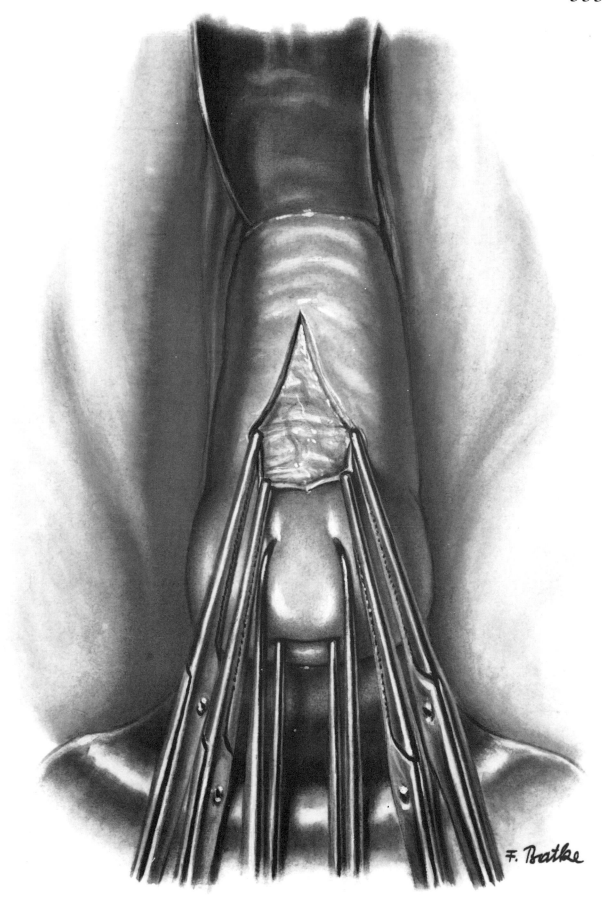

Figure 175. *See legend on opposite page.*

Incision Depth

The depth of the coloptomy incision will depend on the degree of the cystocele. If the cystocele is minimal, the vaginal wall is incised down to the underlying fascia vaginalis, taking care not to injure this tissue. Subsequently, one will dissect laterally between the mucosa and the fascia. This method appears most elegant to the observer because none of the blood vessels coursing in the fascia are opened by it and the operative field remains dry. However, this approach—in which the mucosa is separated from the fascia and the bladder and its covering vaginal fascia are later plicated—is applicable only when a small cystocele is present.

For greater degrees of cystocele the median incision must be made deeper. It is carried through the mucosa and the vaginal fascia in order to open the vesicovaginal space. After the vaginal fascia has been divided, the bladder is exposed; it is also covered by a fas-

Figure 176.

Anterior colporrhaphy. Preparing the operative field for dissection of the right vaginal wall. The midline incision in the anterior vaginal wall has been extended from the portio to just beneath the external urethral meatus. A single clamp placed at the upper wound angle is pulled up by the left assistant's right hand. The left-sided clamps are held in parallel by the left assistant and gently pulled to the side. The right assistant fans out the clamps on the right side with both hands.

See illustration on opposite page.

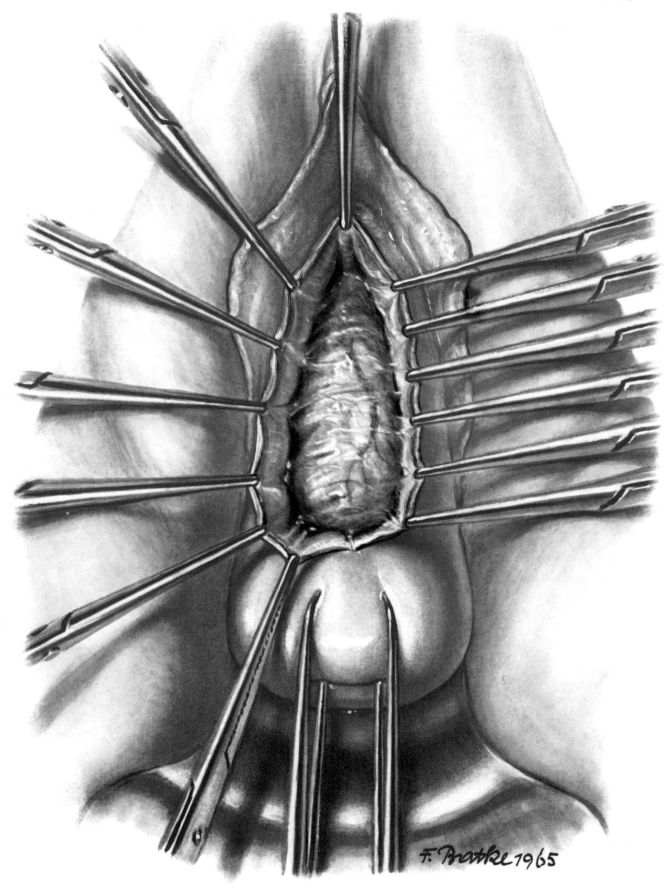

Figure 176. *See legend on opposite page.*

cia. Later, one will dissect between the fascia vaginalis and the fascia vesicalis, separating off the vaginal wall (with mucosa and fascia together) from the bladder and its covering fascia. Dissection between the vaginal fascia and the bladder has the advantage of permitting better mobilization of the bladder once the vesicovaginal space has been opened; also the lower pole of the bladder, which adheres to the cervix by the supravaginal septum, can be dissected free. With a larger cystocele, it is expedient to advance the lower bladder pole to well above the peritoneal reflection.

One of the disadvantages of dissecting between the bladder and the vaginal fascia is the venous bleeding that can occur from damage to the vessels that course in the fascia. This bleeding is always easy to control and must be accepted with a large cystocele because the cystocele has to be elevated, the bladder base and urethral supporting tissues have to be reconstructed and the lower pole of the bladder has to be lifted; in order to accomplish these objectives, the vesicovaginal space must be opened and the supravaginal septum severed.

Figure 177.

Anterior colporrhaphy. Dissecting the right vaginal wall. The right vaginal wound edge is stretched in a fanwise manner. One dissects laterally between the vaginal fascia and the mucosa. The fascia vaginalis remains attached to the vesical fascia on the bladder.

See illustration on opposite page.

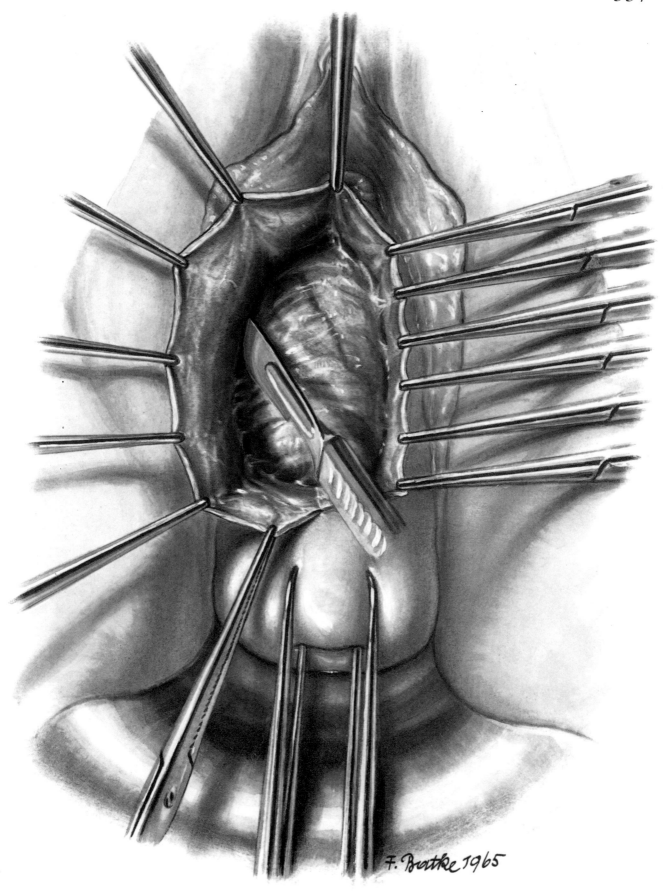

Figure 177. *See legend on opposite page.*

ANTERIOR VAGINOPLASTY WITH MILD CYSTOCELE

After exposing the portio with spatulas, the surgeon grasps the anterior lip of the cervix with two single-toothed tenacula and pulls it forcibly downward. The right assistant lifts and stretches the anterior vaginal wall with a spatula. The incision is begun closely above the portio with a scalpel and is at first extended up only a few centimeters in the midline (Fig. 174). With moderate degrees of descensus, one only divides the vaginal mucosa. The wound edges are held with toothed clamps. The surgeon now relinquishes the tenacula to the left assistant (who holds them in his left hand) and pulls down on the clamps attached to the right vaginal wound edge. The

Figure 178.

Anterior colporrhaphy. Dissecting the left vaginal wall. The right vaginal flap has been dissected. The clamps on the left vaginal wall are fanned out by the left assistant using both hands. The right assistant takes over the midline clamp in his left hand and pulls it upward; in addition, he holds the clamps on the right vaginal wound edge to the side in parallel. The surgeon grasps the bladder and its overlying vesical and vaginal fascias with tissue forceps and pulls medially; sharp dissection is carried out on the left side between the mucosa and the fascia with a scalpel. The better the mucosa is fanned out by traction on the attached clamps, and the more the bladder is pulled medially by the forceps, the easier it is to dissect in the correct layer.

See illustration on opposite page.

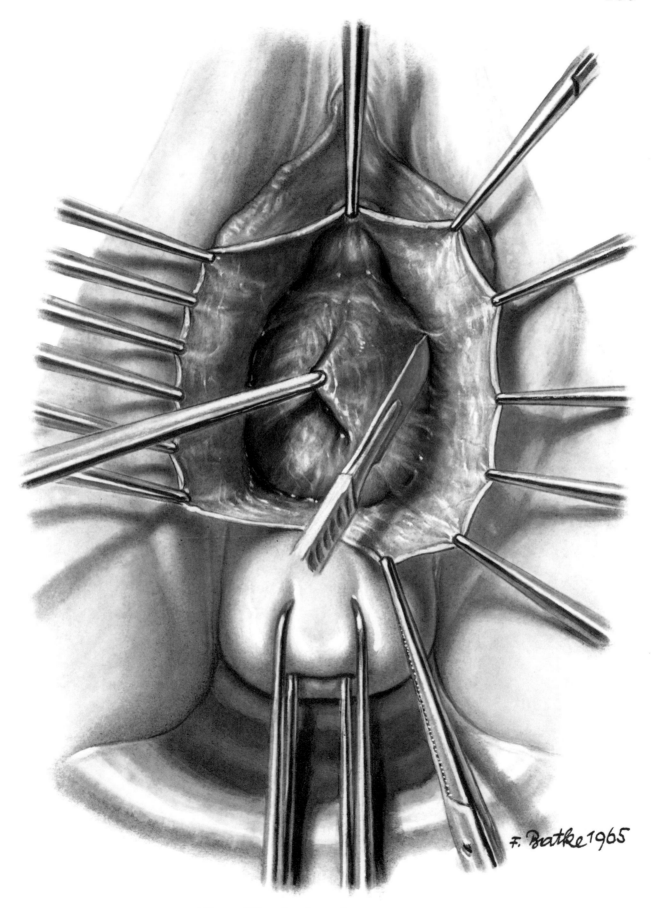

Figure 178.   *See legend on opposite page.*

corresponding clamps on the left side are pulled downward by the left assistant's right hand. The anterior vaginal wall is placed on stretch again by appropriate counterpressure of the anterior spatula (held by the right assistant) (Fig. 175).

The median incision is now extended further upward. Toothed clamps are placed in stepwise fashion on the wound edges. A single clamp is applied at the uppermost wound angle of the median colpotomy incision. By ensuring carefully regulated counterpressure on the vaginal wall, one facilitates the procedure so that it is executed in the proper depth. This is a matter of considerable importance in carrying out the plastic procedure.

Dissecting the Right Vaginal Wall Flap

The right assistant pulls apart the clamps attached to the right side, spreading them fanwise with both hands so that the right vaginal wound edge is smoothly stretched. In order to spread the

Figure 179.

Anterior colporrhaphy. Placing the suburethral purse-string suture. The vaginal wall has been dissected bilaterally, leaving the vaginal and vesical fascias intact. The clamps on the vaginal wound edges are held horizontally by the assistants on either side. The left assistant has taken hold of the uppermost midline clamp with his right hand and is pulling it upward. The paraurethral tissue at the urethrovesical juncture is ligated first, placing the needle on the left side from above down and then on the right side in the same way. While this suture is being tied, the tissues of the bladder neck and urethra are pushed back by tissue forceps held by the right assistant, thus invaginating them.

See illustration on opposite page.

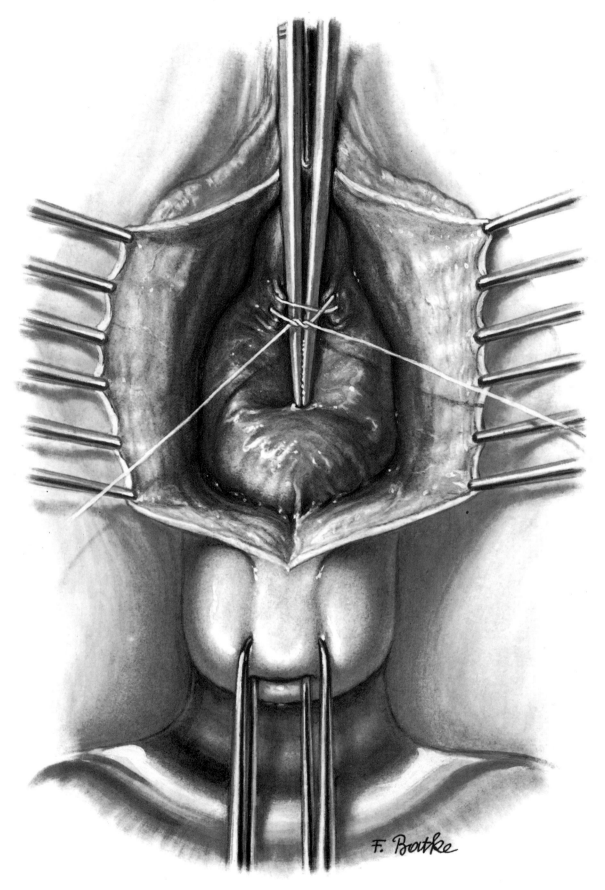

Figure 179. *See legend on opposite page.*

Dissecting the Left Vaginal Wall Flap

Analogous steps are carried out on the left side. The left assistant places the left vaginal wall on stretch by fanning out the attached toothed clamps with both hands; the right assistant retracts the corresponding right-sided clamps to the side, holding them all in parallel, and pulls the uppermost midline clamp upward. The surgeon pushes the bladder medially with a sponge or a toothed tissue forceps, dissecting the left side between the mucosa and the fascia stepwise with a laterally bowed incision (Fig. 178). In this way the bladder is separated from the overlying vagina on the left side.

Plicating the Bladder

After the bladder neck and urethra have been sufficiently prepared, one or two purse-string sutures are placed at the level of the internal urethral orifice (Fig. 179). By means of paraurethral plica-

Figure 181.

Anterior colporrhaphy. Resecting the superfluous vaginal mucosa. The bladder has been plicated; the excess mucosa is being excised elliptically on the right side. To do this, the surgeon pulls down on two of the lowest clamps; the right assistant fans out the upper three clamps and holds back the right labia with a lateral spatula.

See illustration on opposite page.

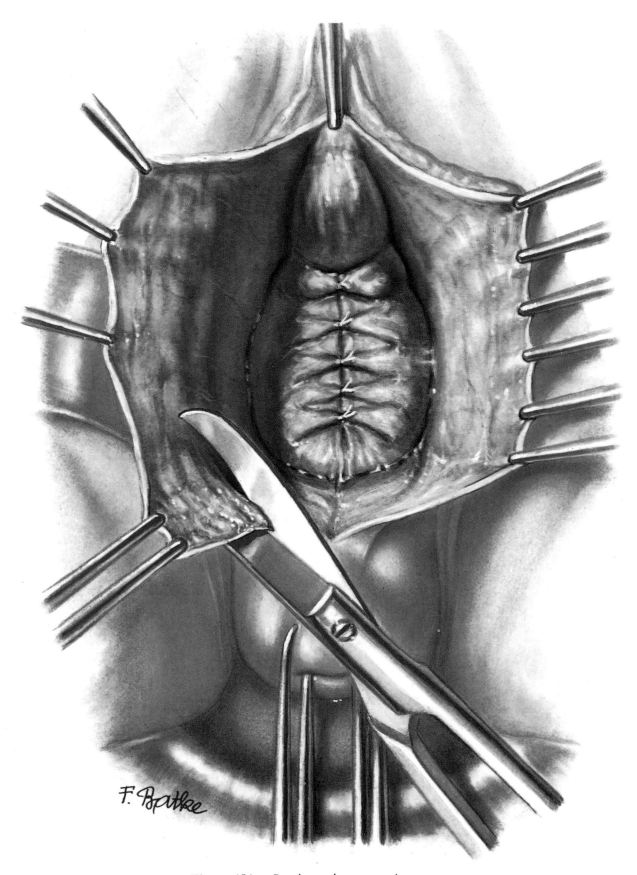

Figure 181.   *See legend on opposite page.*

to plicate the vaginal fascia as far laterally as possible without causing excessive tension to develop in the tissues. The lowest bladder purse-string suture is fixed to the anterior wall of the cervix to form a supplementary "supravaginal septum."

Resecting the Vaginal Wall

Portions of the redundant vaginal flaps are excised from both the right and left sides so that an elliptical resection of the anterior vaginal wall is accomplished (Fig. 181).

Closing the Colpotomy Wound

After the vaginal wall has been trimmed, the edges of the vaginal incision are joined in the midline by interrupted horizontal mattress catgut sutures. The following technique is advisable for closure because the distal vaginal wound edges will usually retract after the first one or two sutures have been placed at the upper angle, obscuring exposure and making further coaptation difficult. After two sutures have been inserted at the uppermost wound angle, two like sutures are placed to join the vaginal edges at the lowest angle. By simultaneously pulling the upper sutures upward and the lower sutures downward, one exposes the vaginal wound to view and facilitates suturing the edges together (Figs. 182 and 183). One proceeds then to suture from the caudal end up to the cranial; in this way one can pull on each caudally placed suture in turn to retract the wound edge progressively forward until the entire wound is in full view.

Figure 183.

Anterior colporrhaphy. Closing the median colpotomy. The anterior vaginal wound is closed. Its typical S-shaped course is illustrated.

See illustration on opposite page.

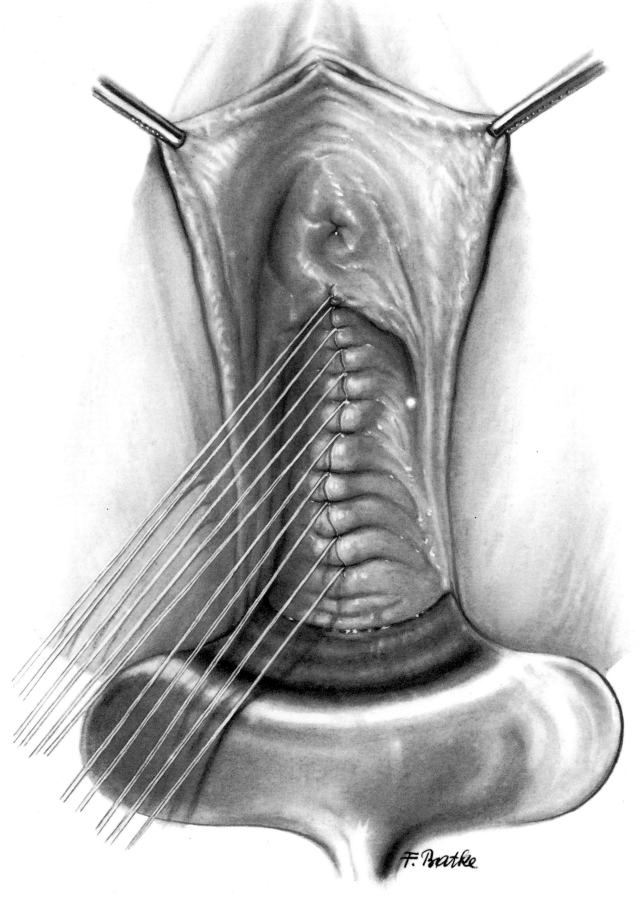

Figure 183. *See legend on opposite page.*

ANTERIOR VAGINOPLASTY IN EXTENSIVE CYSTOCELE

In the patient with an advanced cystocele, the median colpotomy incision is carried down to a depth that divides both vaginal mucosa and fascia. Thus one opens the vesicovaginal space so that the bladder with its investing fascia is visualized. The bladder is then mobilized laterally by dissecting between the vesical fascia and the vaginal fascia (Fig. 184).

In the course of this dissection, it is readily apparent that the separation of the vesical and vaginal fascias is accomplished much more easily near the portio than near the bladder neck or over the

Figure 184.

Anterior colporrhaphy with extensive cystocele. Dissection of the vaginal wall fascial flap on the left side. The midline colpotomy involved severing the vaginal wall through the vascular fascia vaginalis down to the fascia vesicalis. The right vaginal wall flap is completely separated from the bladder. The clamps on the left vaginal wound edge are fanned out by the left assistant with both hands. The right assistant lifts the single clamp at the upper angle with his left hand while he pulls the clamps attached to the right vaginal wound edge to the side with his other hand, holding them in parallel. The surgeon pushes the bladder medially with a sponge held in a clamp and dissects laterally between the vesical and vaginal fascias. Anteriorly at the bladder neck and urethra, a portion of the vaginal fascia is densely interwoven with the bladder fascia that is left attached to the bladder so as to avoid injuries.

See illustration on opposite page.

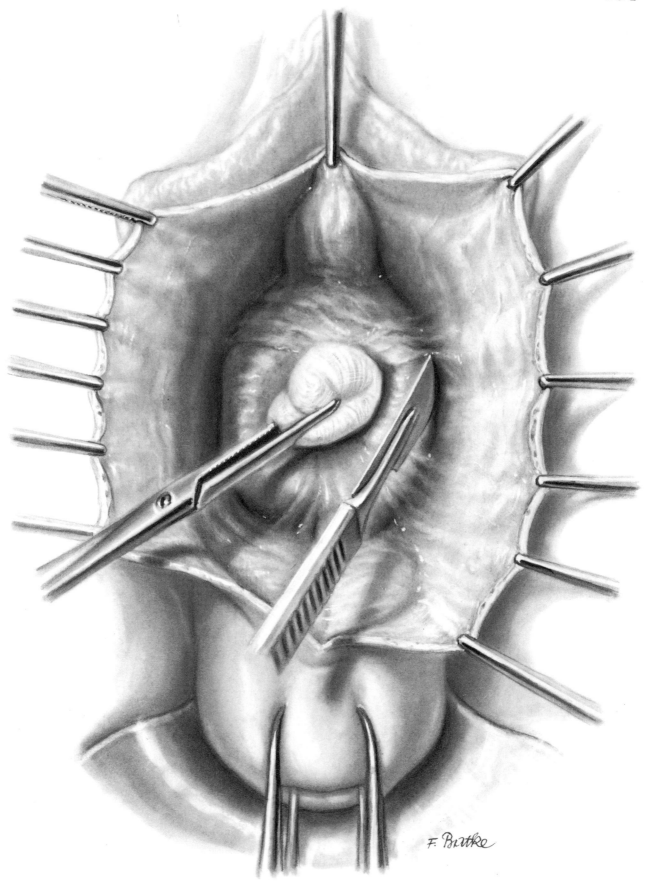

Figure 184. *See legend on opposite page.*

urethra. This is explained by the anatomic fact that the fascia overlying the bladder neck and urethra is very closely intertwined with the vaginal fascia; in the vicinity of the bladder neck they blend into a connective tissue layer that extends to the region of the upper third of the urethra (septum urethrovaginale). One should take particular care in this area to carry out the dissection sharply with a scalpel in order to avoid injuring the bladder or the urethra. One should dissect only the vaginal mucosa in this location, leaving a portion of the vaginal fascia attached to the bladder fascia.

The vaginal fascia and mucosa are extensively dissected bilaterally caudad to the bladder neck. Then the lower pole of the bladder, which is fixed to the anterior cervix by the supravaginal septum, is widely mobilized (Fig. 185). One severs the septum to open the vesicocervical space and then advances the bladder to a point above the anterior peritoneal reflection. The descended bladder is freed up laterally and caudally. One or two suburethral purse-string

Figure 185.

Anterior colporrhaphy with extensive cystocele. Dividing the supravaginal septum. The vaginal wall fascial flaps have been dissected bilaterally. A part of the vaginal fascia was left adherent to the bladder in the region of the bladder neck. The left assistant pulls the tenacula down with his left hand and the right assistant similarly pulls the uppermost wound angle clamp gently upward; the lateral clamps are held in parallel and pulled laterally by both assistants. The surgeon lifts the lower pole of the bladder with tissue forceps and severs the stretched connective tissue bands of the supravaginal septum close to the cervix with scissors, pointing the tips of the scissors toward the cervix.

See illustration on opposite page.

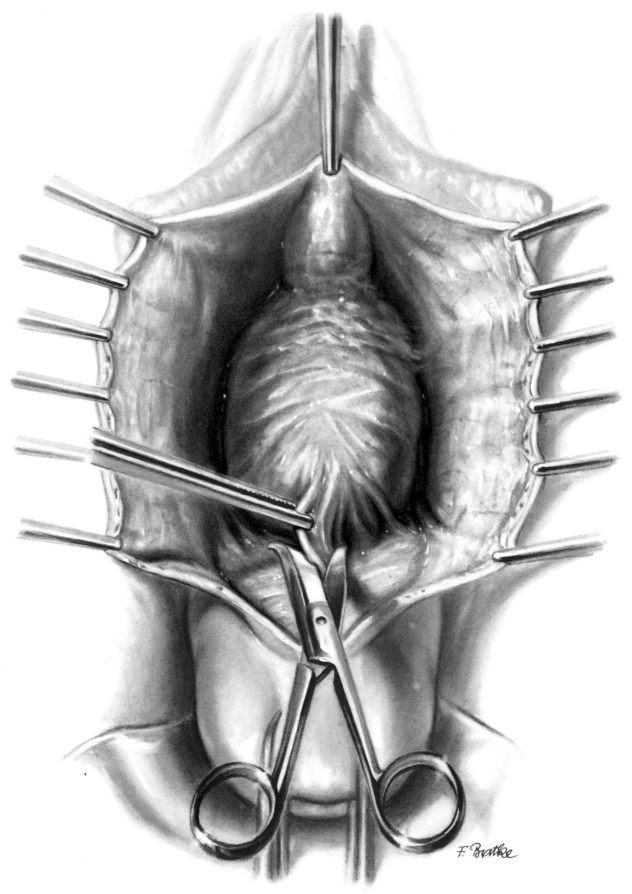

Figure 185. *See legend on opposite page.*

sutures are now applied. The rest of the mobilized bladder is plicated with a half-purse-string suture (Figs. 186 and 187) or a row of sagittal mattress sutures. After this has been done, the bladder pillars can be joined in the midline and fixed to the anterior cervix. Resection of superfluous vaginal mucosa is carried out, together with closure of the colpotomy wound, as previously described.

Technical Problems

1. Incorrect depth of incision is possible in performing the median colpotomy. With a large cystocele, the colpotomy must cut through both mucosa and fascia in the lower two-thirds of the incision in order to reach into the vesicovaginal space. Only if this space is opened will it be feasible to mobilize the lower pole of the descended bladder extensively. Near the external urethral meatus

Figure 186.

Anterior colporrhaphy with extensive cystocele. Plicating the bladder. The vaginal wall flaps have been dissected bilaterally and the lower bladder pole advanced up to the peritoneal reflection after the supravaginal septum was dissected and the vesicocervical space opened. Remnants of the dissected supravaginal septum are recognizable still attached to the anterior wall of the cervix. A purse-string suture is already in place suburethrally at the bladder neck. For further plication of the mobilized bladder, a half-purse-string suture is placed, beginning on the left side at the site of the first suburethral suture and reaching caudally to the lower bladder pole; it is then continued on the right side upward to the knotted suburethral purse-string suture. The bladder is invaginated with tissue forceps before the suture is tied.

See illustration on opposite page.

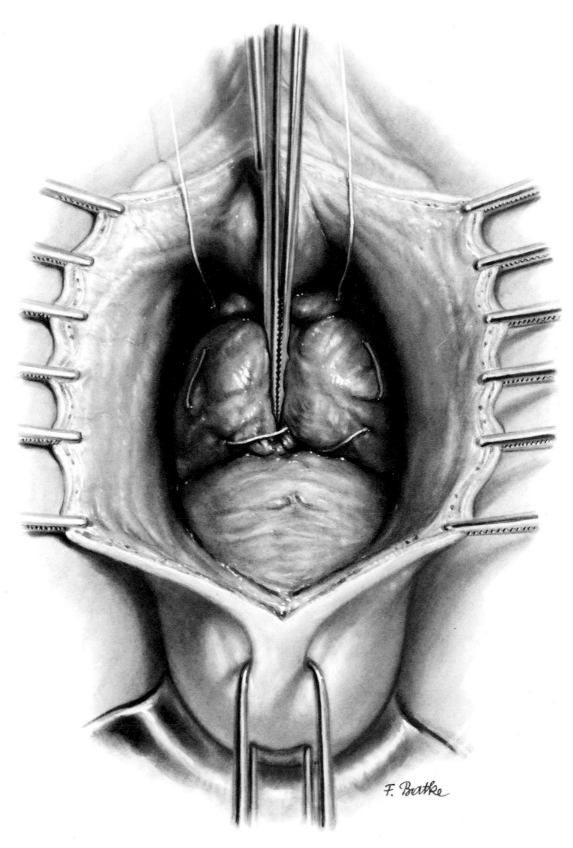

Figure 186. *See legend on opposite page.*

the colpotomy need only incise the mucosa because the vaginal fascia here is intimately interlaced with the bladder fascia and they are inseparable. An incision that is carried too deeply in this site would injure the bladder neck or the anterior wall of the urethra.

2. The median colpotomy may be extended too far upward or downward. The upper wound should end about 1 cm. caudad to the urethral meatus; if it should go higher, damage to the anterior urethra may result. The lower wound ought to end at the point where the loose vaginal mucosa meets the fixed mucosa of the portio.

3. If the toothed clamps attached to the vaginal flaps are not retracted uniformly and fanned out properly during the dissection of the mucosa or the fascia, separating the layers is made more difficult. Also the vaginal mucosa can be perforated as a consequence.

4. The wrong tissue layers may be entered or the vagina cut through if the assistants retract the vaginal flaps too far laterally so that they are bent over, even though the attached clamps are being fanned out properly. This may happen despite care exerted in gently stroking the tissues with the scalpel blade. It can generally be avoided by ensuring that the assistant does not pull too strongly in a lateral direction upon the fanned-out clamps (he should retract instead with a more sagittal pull). Simultaneously, the surgeon should deflect the bladder medially with tissue forceps.

Figure 187.

Anterior colporrhaphy with extensive cystocele. View of operative field after plicating the mobilized bladder. The suburethral and bladder plication sutures have been placed and tied. These not only have plicated the bladder, but have elevated it as well. The lower extent of the peritoneal reflection is seen.

See illustration on opposite page.

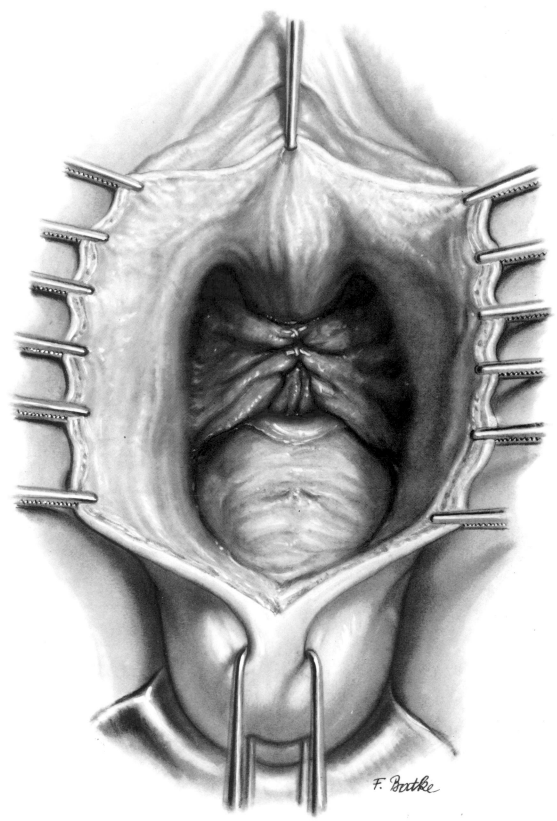

Figure 187. *See legend on opposite page.*

5. In patients with vaginal prolapse, the vaginal wall is usually thickened and its component layers are poorly formed. Under these circumstances, separation of the vaginal fascia flap from the bladder should always be done by sharp dissection, never bluntly.

6. The vaginal wall at the upper end of the median incision may be insufficiently mobilized. In those cases with urethrocele it is especially important that extensive lateral dissection be done in the area of the bladder neck and urethra so that enough periurethral and perivesical tissue is exposed for later plication. Because of the dense interconnection here between the bladder and vaginal fascias, dissection must be done sharply with a scalpel and the vaginal mucosa separated from its fascia with small stepwise cuts. For this the left assistant has to lift the upper angle clamp with moderate force precisely in the midline. The surgeon must direct the blade of the scalpel so that it is slanted laterally, thus avoiding injury to the urethra. He always dissects close to the vaginal wall and leaves the vaginal fascia in this area attached to the fascia overlying the urethra and the bladder neck. After correctly dissecting in this region, one can recognize the urethrovesical transition forming a distinctive angulation at the internal urethral orifice where the urethra exits from the bladder.

7. If dissection is carried too far laterally in the upper third of the vaginal wall, the lateral aspects of the space of Retzius are entered. Some of the many veins draining the bladder may be injured here. The resulting hemorrhage cannot be staunched by the vaginal tamponade that will be done later, but has to be stopped by means of ligation. The needle for such ligatures should always be pointed laterally away from the urethra toward the pubic arch; it must not be applied in the reverse direction or the urethra may be punctured.

8. Overly enthusiastic dissection laterally close to the descending ramus of the pubis may cause venous bleeding that, if not too heavy, can be stilled later by vaginal tamponade; if heavy, however, the source of the bleeding must be ligated.

9. In the case of a markedly descended bladder, the lower pole of the bladder and perhaps even the distal part of the bladder pillar (which is laterally stretched) has to be well mobilized and pushed far upwards. When done properly this displaces the ureters coursing in the bladder pillars so that they are out of danger of being incorporated into the bladder plication purse-string sutures. Nevertheless, because the hazard of ureteral damage persists, the purse-string sutures used to join the bladder pillars in the midline should not be placed too far laterally.

10. If the supravaginal septum is divided incompletely in association with extensive bladder descent, the lower pole of the bladder cannot be adequately mobilized and the bladder cannot be advanced

up to its original location. To avoid this problem it is occasionally necessary to incise the stretched bladder pillars near the cervix. Venous bleeding that may result is easily controlled.

11. The excess vaginal mucosa can be too extensively resected, especially in its lateral aspects. As a consequence of this error, coaptation of the vaginal wound edges will be done with unacceptable tension that may lead to postoperative dehiscence. Even if the colpotomy wound can just be closed without apparent tension on the mattress sutures, it is still possible that too much of the vaginal wall has been resected; this situation will be recognized only at the end of the procedure. After reconstruction of the perineum, the vaginal introitus may barely admit two fingers; this will cause coital problems. If less of the anterior vaginal wall is resected, the vaginal width will be adequate despite the perineal repair. It should be possible, therefore, to unite the anterior vaginal wound edges without tension. The amount of superfluous vaginal wall to be resected depends on the extent of descensus, but in general it is better to excise too little than too much. It is not essential for correcting urinary incontinence that the excess vaginal wall be resected precisely; more important are the correct placement of the suburethral and bladder plication sutures, reconstruction of the relaxed pelvic floor by uniting the freed eges of the levators and rebuilding the perineum.

12. The cut edges of the vaginal fascia must be sutured with broad ligatures during closure of the anterior colpotomy wound so that bleeding from severed vessels located in the fascia is stopped. However, it is just as important not to strangulate the tissue with closely spaced sutures that will make the thin flaps become necrotic. Furthermore, it is important that any postoperative blood seepage be allowed to escape between the sutures.

13. The anterior colpotomy wound should be closed with interrupted 00 chromic catgut sutures; a continuous suture would shorten the vagina. Moreover, the vaginal wound edges can be coapted better by interrupted sutures than by a continuous suture.

14. The vaginal canal may be made too narrow by the anterior colporrhaphy and colpoperineoplasty procedures (it should be able to accommodate at least two fingers). If one finds at the conclusion of the perineal reconstruction that sexual intercourse will probably not be possible as a result of the excessive vaginal narrowing, it is advisable to make small lengthwise releasing incisions at 5 and 7 o'clock, respectively, in the lateral vaginal walls and then suture them transversely. This technique is not ideal, but it does enlarge the vaginal lumen without having to cut the sutures that have just been placed for purposes of constructing the perineum and alleviating incontinence.

OVERLAPPING THE FASCIA

With a very extensive cystocele, it is sometimes advantageous to overlap the fascia. In this procedure the median longitudinal incision is carried down through the anterior vaginal mucosa and fascia into the vesicovaginal space. The fascial flaps are developed bilaterally, dissecting them free of the bladder, its covering fascia and the urethra. Now the flaps are divided into their two component lamellae so that the fascia vaginalis is separated from the mucosa.

Figure 188.

Anterior colporrhaphy. Overlapping the fascia. Separating both components of the left vaginal wall flap. The median colpotomy incision in the anterior vaginal wall has been carried through the vaginal mucosa and fascia down to the bladder fascia. Both flaps are dissected from the bladder (the bladder is covered by the vesical fascia). The right vaginal flap has already been split into its two layers by separation of the vaginal fascia from the mucosa (for purposes of visualization of the structures the clamps are not shown here). The left assistant fans out the left vaginal wall clamps. On the left side, dissection is being carried out between the mucosa and the fascia vaginalis, separating both flaps into two tissue layers for purposes of overlapping.

See illustration on opposite page.

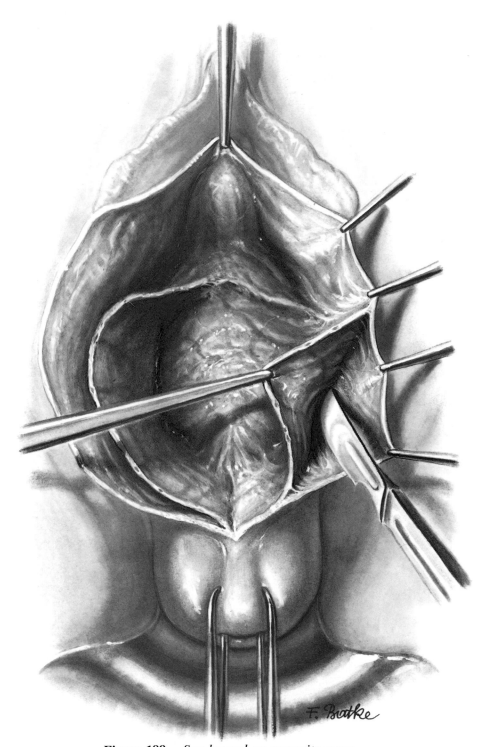

Figure 188.   *See legend on opposite page.*

The external homogeneous layer corresponding to the vaginal mucosa is recognized and can be distinguished from the inner vaginal fascia layer in which blood vessels are located (Fig. 188). By separating the vaginal mucosa from the fascia, two sets of superimposable flaps are formed (one mucosal and one fascial flap on each side).

After the supravaginal septum has been severed, the bladder can be well mobilized. Next, one begins to place the previously described invagination sutures in the region of the urethrovesical juncture. This is followed by similar sutures in the posterior sector of the bladder floor; these plicate the bladder wall and fascia vesicalis by means of a sagittal row of horizontal mattress sutures or a purse-string suture.

Figure 189.

Anterior colporrhaphy. Overlapping the fascia. Fixing the right vaginal flap to the left side. After the supravaginal septum was divided, the lower bladder pole was extensively mobilized. At the urethrovesical juncture, an invaginating suture has been placed and the rest of the bladder has also been plicated with a purse-string suture. Both vaginal flaps are split into their component lamellae of mucosa and fascia. Partial resection of the superfluous vaginal fascia is done and the medial edge of the right flap is laid to the left over the plicated bladder in the furrow between the bladder and the left flap of fascia vaginalis, where it is fixed with interrupted sutures.

See illustration on opposite page.

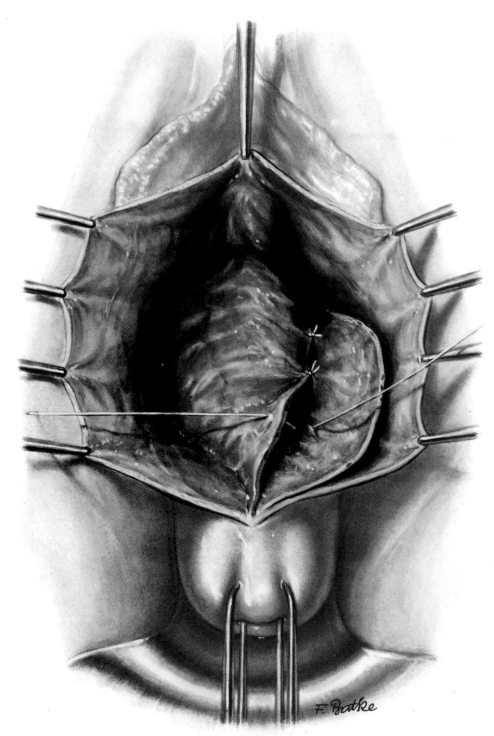

Figure 189.   *See legend on opposite page.*

At this time the right fascial flap is laid to the left over the plicated bladder base; it is sutured down with interrupted sutures in the furrow between the bladder and the left flap of the fascia (Fig. 189). Then the left fascial flap is lapped over the right side and affixed by suturing in the furrow between the mucosa and the fascial flap (Fig. 190). Thus both fascial flaps are placed so that they overlap each other upon the plicated bladder. Elliptical excision of the superfluous part of the vaginal mucosa and coaptation of the vaginal wound with interrupted sutures is then done as described above.

Figure 190.

Anterior colporrhaphy. Overlapping the fascia. Fixing the left vaginal flap to the right side. The right fascial flap is already folded to the left over the plicated bladder and fixed with interrupted sutures. The left flap is folded to the right over the previously anchored right flap and its edge is fixed into the furrow between the mucosa and the base of the right vaginal fascia with interrupted sutures. In this way, both flaps are overlapped.

See illustration on opposite page.

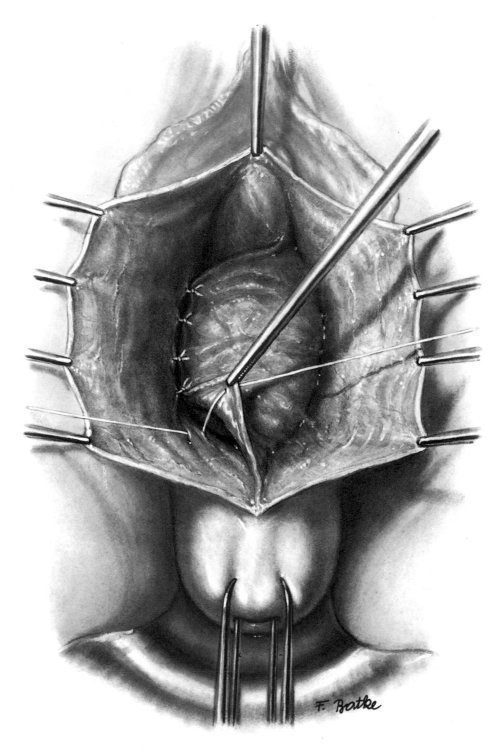

Figure 190. *See legend on opposite page.*